What's Behind Your Belly Button?

A PSYCHOLOGICAL PERSPECTIVE OF THE INTELLIGENCE OF HUMAN NATURE AND GUT INSTINCT

By Martha Char Love and Robert W. Sterling

DEDICATION

This book is dedicated to the youth who, in the 1950s and the 1960s, tried to awaken the culture to the feeling that something far more important than material waste and worldly possessions would lead us as a nation away from war and self destruction. "Give peace a chance" and "love" in its many forms would bring diverse human differences together and, like for the authors of this book, there was no accurate image available to make it happen. Since there was no clear guide and the deep feeling of emptiness could not be filled with what understanding was available, there was not sufficient energy available to keep the action alive. However, much has happened since then in our understanding of human nature that we hope will bring us closer to the goal that was then just a feeling in the late Sixties. The feeling is very much alive and the stuff to make it happen requires a simple adaptation of our thinking along with that same feeling. We wish you balance of Self-Control and Self-Acceptance in your lives, and please pass it along to the children.

"For the great enemy of truth is very often not the lie—deliberate, contrived, and dishonest—but the myth—persistent, persuasive, and unrealistic. Too often we hold fast to the clichés of our forbears. We subject all facts to a prefabricated set of interpretations. We enjoy the comfort of opinion without the discomfort of thought."

(John F Kennedy, Yale Commencement, 1962)

TABLE OF CONTENTS

Preface 13

Introduction.. 23

Chapter One:

Development of the Concept of Reflection

on Gut Instincts... 27

    The Purpose:

    Reassessing the Meaning Of Experience........................ 34

    Spontaneous Sharing of Instinctive Feelings:

    The Meaningful Use of Time.. 37

Chapter Two:

Medical Breakthrough Supports the Gut

as a Center of Intelligence 41

    The World of the Enteric Nervous System...................... 43

    Conclusions on Gershon's Research............................ 46

    The World of the Fetus Found to Begin in the Gut 47

    Fetal Construction Schedule:

    Fertilization to Birth—9 Months 48

    Conclusions on Fetal Development 50

Chapter Three:

The Impact of Experience:

The Universal Principles of Feelings................................. 51

    A Process of Self-Awareness.. 54

(Chapter Three Continued)

Caring for Instinctual Feelings.. 60

The Meaningful Use of Time... 62

Anatomy of Feelings.. 64

Levels of Feeling.. 70

Becoming Aware of Instinctive Feelings.......................... 71

Structured Awareness of Feelings 76

    Hostility 77

    Guilt... 80

    Fear 83

    Joy.. 85

When caring Exists 88

Chapter Four:

A New Image of Human Nature 95

    On the Threshold of a Renaissance............................. 95

    Basic Human Needs... 99

    Needed: A New Myth for Humanity

    that Reduces Stress 101

    The New Functional Image of Humanity 104

    Questioning Human Nature

    and the Gut Decision... 111

Chapter Five:

The Development of the Somatic Reflection Process

and a New School of Gut Psychology 115

    Finding the Source of Inner Conflict and Stress........... 116

(Chapter Five Continued)
The MBTI and the Development
of the Somatic Reflection Process 119
Reading Life Backwards.. 124
The Feeling of Emptiness and Fullness
in the Gut 126
Our Instinctual Needs 133
Principles Underlying the Technique
of the Somatic Reflection Process 140
    Centering on the Feelings of Unresolved Issues........ 141
    Becoming Conscious of Inner Needs
    through the Somatic Reflection Process 143

Chapter Six:
Facilitating the Somatic Reflection Process 147
    Three Types of Facilitation............................. 147
        The Somatic Reflection Process with a Facilitator.... 148
        The Somatic Reflection Process
        with an Imaginary Facilitator.................... 150
        The Somatic Reflection Process
        with an Inner Facilitator......................... 151
    Being Attuned as a Facilitator:
    Empty Mind—Full Belly................................ 152
    A Protocol for The Somatic Reflection Process 155
        Identifying the Unresolved Issue and Feeling 157
        Reflecting Backwards in Time with Feelings........... 159
        Finding the Awareness of the
        Rejection of Inner Feelings and Needs.................. 161

(Chapter Six Continued)
Connecting the Feelings of the Past
to the Present Life Issue 164

Chapter Seven:
A Research Exploration on the
Personal Value of the Somatic Reflection Process 165
   Increased Somatic Awareness 166
     Feeling Better 166
     Increase of Awareness of Feelings in the Body 167
   Increased insights 168
     New Perspective 168
     Increased Awareness of Inner Needs 170
   Increased Self-Acceptance 171
   Somatic Reflection Process of
   Researcher Subject: Cindy 172
   Somatic Reflection Process of
   Researcher Subject: Sara 182
   Concluding Remarks 189

Chapter Eight:
Nature's Way 191
   Neuroscience Changes our Way of Viewing
   Ourselves and Our Relationship to Others 194
   Intimacy and Instinctual Gut Responses 199
   The Language of the Gut: ME, MYSELF, AND I 201
   Mobility and the Gut 202
   Adaptability and the Gut 204

(Chapter Eight Continued)

Evolution and the Gut 205

Intuition and the Gut 207

The Maturing of Science Ushers in a

New Image of Human Nature 208

Chapter Nine:

A New Psychology of Gut Instinct 213

The Voice of the Gut 215

Gut Experience 219

Problem Solving and Gut Instincts 223

Renaissance: Freedom and Recognition

of Instinctual Feeling Responses 227

Chapter Ten:

The New Image of Human Nature In Education 231

The Learning Process 232

It Takes a Licken and Keeps On Ticken 234

Applications of New Image to Education 235

Ideals for Education 238

Letter on Education to President Obama 242

Farm to Factory 255

The Analog of Discovery 257

Puberty and Instinctual Needs

Affecting the Learning Process 260

Incarceration: A New Reclamation Project

of Human Life   268

Conclusions on Education   269

Chapter Eleven:

The New Image of Human Nature and Dis-ease 275

The Voice of the Gut and The Cure of Dis-ease 275

Distinguishing the "You Cells"and "Not You Cells" 282

The Somatic Reflection Process
as a Medical Intervention 288

Identifying Elements of the
Somatic Depth Process For Medical Study 291

The Six Phases of Somatic Depth Process 293

Conclusions 296

Chapter Twelve:

The New Image: Our Gut as a Dependable

Center of Reference 299

Authors' Notes and References 303

Further Definition of Some Terms Used 310

References 315

About the Authors 327

ACKNOWLEDGMENTS

I had a good talk with myself this morning so I feel much better now. I decided that I have full control myself and that there was at least one person who could accept my way of life. So here is my latest effort.

PREFACE

In the '70s, we worked as both counselors and instructors in a large community college, Santa Fe Community College (SFCC), in Gainesville Florida. It was a very different time in the field of education than it is today. Experimentation of learning processes in the classroom was not only possible, but also encouraged—at least in many schools around the country. It was an era prior to the deluge of lawsuits that closed the doors to experiencing the spontaneity in the classroom necessary for the exploration into the inner worlds of human feelings. Some very forward thinking educators, including Dr. Joe Fordyce, Dr. Terry O'Banion, and Dr. Bob Shepack, to whom we will be forever grateful for the educational environment they cultivated, set up SFCC as an experimental humanistic oriented school. Their effort was to affect change in the process of learning in the Jr. College, in the 1960s, which created an environment of intuitive, in-depth, problem solving. We took them seriously at the time, and, with the help of modern medical research, today we have further validation of its pervasive value to our modern culture.

We were fortunate enough to be there at the right time in human history to engage in an experience that brought on our discovery of the true inner nature of human beings and ground breaking clinical experience in the field of psychology involving the gut response center. Since we were instrumental in establishing and operating a career guidance center for the college, much of the early material in this book is our day-to-day experience in both the career guidance center and Behavioral Science classes, in which we were teaching, and in which learning about the inner nature of the person was being discovered and shared. We found, that in order to deal with the problems of career choice, people needed to first deal with the understanding of the authentic

Self and it's concepts. From this approach, we developed a methodology for access to the inner instinctive processes, where the impact of life's experience resides, and where the energy towards individual goals is found—not in the goals obtained from external authorities. Such an impact of experience provides the energy, the life drive for the adult, which is closely related to the excitement experienced early as a child.

The process by which inner awareness of the Self is experienced is the theme of this book. This process is learned through the person's own experience of himself, not by way of formal education. It is available to all persons who seek to become aware of the Self that lies fallow in the instincts of all human beings. It is, therefore, a process of becoming more aware of what we already, subconsciously or consciously, know about ourselves.

We have developed a functional model for Self-awareness by the individual rather than an observational model for a helping profession. In holding and supporting this functional point of view, we are concerned only with the inner experiential Self-awareness point of view of the person. This task is the essence of the problem for each individual life in experience. Each person is faced with keeping track of his own inner feelings about himself while dealing with the outer judgments of others about his observable behavior.

There seems to be many counter productive folkways and morays that conflict with instinctive human needs. These habits of 'thoughtless logic', conceived long before our time, have produced images of human nature destructive to the health and welfare of all ages. We cautiously discuss some of these issues relative to common knowledge now available.

In this book, we have tried to include both material that is experiential and feeling, as well as material that explains our research from a more logical, even at times an academic point of, view. The following is a summary of material presented chapter by chapter:

Chapter One. We introduce the reader to the discovery of the gut intelligence responses in our early clinical studies, as well as to the history and development of the Somatic Reflection Process (SRP). Much of this is a revision from our earlier writings, *Borne of the Human Family*, 1976, which we had published at Santa Fe Community College, Gainesville, FL, and used as a text for the Behavioral Sciences classes we were teaching. Our first book, *Borne of the Human Family*, is an explicit model and a methodology, introducing the Somatic Reflection Process, which makes a clear statement of the human ability in socialization: "how to get close and not get lost".

At the time of our counseling assignment, there probably had never been as pervasive and as deep a display of public feeling over a previous war. The Viet Nam war made no sense to anyone particularly, to the youth of this country who were conscripted to fight it—there was no creditable logic to support it.

We offer this reflection of the time to suggest to many of you who were not present at that time, that the '70s was a time when there had been no affective emotional recovery from the war, and drug relief had set in, as an attempt to numb the upper brain and quell the emotions. This was a time of confusion for everyone, which, in one sense, made most of the counseling 'tools' with which we had to work, obsolete— making the task more difficult. But, in another sense, this unique situation made the students more eager to discuss their feelings, which encouraged us to dig deeper into our own feelings; all of which made the task more rewarding and more productive.

Chapter Two. We introduce two major bodies of neurological research, which have emerged in the last two decades and is significant to our work and validates our findings concerning the gut response as a center of intelligence. The physiology of the source of somatic-feelings remained a mystery to us in our early study of human nature and gut instinctive feelings in the 1970s. We knew that the feelings, with which we were working, were stored in the gut as pure feelings without logical thinking attached, but we had no image of the specific source of the feelings in the human anatomy. It was not until recent years when we first read of some important neurological research, that a clear physiological connection was made and we understood it to be a validation of our early work.

Chapter Three. This chapter introduces the concepts and principles transposed from the medical view to a basic psychological—behavioral significance.

We demonstrate, as a result of our clinical experience and the results of the cited neurological research, that we are dealing with a quality of intelligence common and available to all human beings. We have found that when these two centers of guidance, head and gut, are in balance, they can offer greater satisfaction and stability to emotional experiences to both individuals and groups in all enterprises of life. We explore how somatic modalities like the Somatic Reflection Process are successful in reducing stress and may be employed as a healing process to reduce dis-ease. It is the purpose of our presentation to identify images of the head and gut that will help individuals discover awareness and balance between these two centers of intelligence, and, thereby, achieve a higher standard of health and satisfaction in their lives, and bring on a Renaissance to the human family awareness. When the individual achieves a unity of mind and body and the individual's instinctive inner needs are met, the person and culture benefit from a higher standard of ethics, morality, health and quality of life.

Chapter Four. It is from the awareness of two centers of intelligence in the human being and in Gershon's medical research and discovery of our two brains, that we view a new image of human nature necessary to take us into the 21st century and beyond. We describe the experience that understanding this new image of human nature gives to us and the self-awareness this knowledge brings in ourselves and in others to give us the perspective necessary to thrive as individuals during this difficult era of change we are presently living in, and thus assisting the growth of our humanity in making effective changes in our societies. The referenced changes include an essential greater awareness of the inner human nature, basic instinctive human needs, (Self-control and Self-acceptance), and the understanding of the need for balance between our thinking and feeling intelligence centers.

We present a view of the development of a fetus and its development of the two intelligence centers— the thinking and gut brains, as well as the schedule of construction of the fetus and these centers, and its completion at birth. We also deal with the affect of the fact that only after birth, the construction of the head brain fully develops its tools (sight, sound, taste, touch, and smell), and discuss how these tools are of adequate quality depending on the stimulation of the environments to which the new born is exposed.

We show that there is the built-in system in the human being capable of self-control and care for others without the influence of any outside control. We see these characteristics as the result of stability furnished by the presence of the two centers of intelligence working together providing self regulating feed-back with the upper brain, focused on the outside world, and the gut brain focused on the inner body functions—digestion, and energy generation. We leave no question about, which is the most dependable center of intelligence. It is with Chapter Four that we prepare the reader for the understanding that the knowledge of the intelligence of the enteric nervous system is the bases for the development of a new Gut Psychology.

Chapter Five. As you will see, the Somatic Reflection Process (SRP) is designed to purge the disturbance aspect of misunderstood experiences of the past, from continuing to distort experiences of the present, in order to increase confidence of movement into the future, by reflecting back to the source with feelings. This result requires the new image of human nature with its pure feeling, the elimination of pure logic of the upper brain, and the relationship between the two centers of intelligence—feeling and thinking—working in concert. In this chapter we define the new image of humanity with intelligence in the head and a second center of intelligence in the gut

Chapter Six. This chapter is used to demonstrate and explain the intricacies of the methodology and protocol of the Somatic Reflection Process (SRP). Onc of the authors facilitated the SRP in an achedemic setting, in a research study with individual colleagues in her Masters Program in Depth Psychology in 2005 at Sonoma State University—the reflection is verbatim.

Chapter Seven. This chapter is devoted to the evaluation of the results of Chapter Six. These results demonstrate the responses of the research participants in the SRP study and their gains of increased somatic awareness—including feeling better with more adequate sleep and relief of tension in the body; increased insights of problems and inner issues with a new perspective and awareness of inner needs, and increased feelings of self-acceptance—a clearer understanding of them selves.

Chapter Eight. This chapter, *Natures Way*, will probably be the most difficult for the reader, the strangest aspect of all to understand and accept. We have taken the results of experience and research—psychological and medical—and formed that material into a new image of human nature—an image of dual intelligences. In this new perspective, we have discovered the patterns of Nature—an inclusive paradigm of Nature's way that includes other sciences; then we intuit a coherent set of behaviors to be expected from humans with two brains instead of just one (from the boundary conditions permitted by the new paradigm). This was written in the years after our work together at SFCC and is taken from our two minds reflecting independently over a period of thirty-seven years on the same subject—human nature, then comparing notes and arriving at the same conclusions after the years of separation.

Chapter Nine. Underlying the material in this chapter is the awareness of a change in psychology, a change from the disruptive psychology of external guessing of the meaning of human behavior, to an inner psychology of a dependable center of essential intelligence, which when consciously used is a stabilizing influence to human behavior. This center, located in the gut, contains the architecture for the Human design, the DNA, and the Human building plan, the RNA for the Human organism. It is in this same area that the animal instincts are found. However, the characteristics of the instincts have been miss used and miss understood, in the past, named as an evil aspect of the Human personality. The results of neurological and psychological research over the past fifty years now indicate that the consciously learned use of the gut intelligence provides behavior patterns that will lead to Self-Control and Self-Acceptance—with no need for external control or behavioral instructions. The combination of the Main brain with its central nervous system, and the ancient Animal Brain with its somatic, enteric nervous system in the inner body—in the gut—and the constant dialog between them provides a self-correcting feedback system, which regulates the behavioral qualities of the organism when consciously cultivated—preferably in early youth.

We examine the benefits of discovery of the second-brain voice of feeling in the gut, as opposed to the exclusive use of the upper brain in the head with its powerful thinking sensory skills. This combination of inside—outside intelligence balance provides for intellectual growth: problem solving, mobility, adaptability, intuition, and reflective clearing of past disruptive miss understandings—that interfere in the present—with emotional guilt, bursts of hostility in the present, and fear of the future.

We discuss some of the institutional positions with its barriers to the dramatic changes that the educated use of the second brain imposes on the society. It appears that a conscious, balanced use of the two centers of intelligence has never been allowed to emerge in human history—for reasons not absolutely clear we haven't used the brains we were born with.

Chapter Ten. This chapter discusses the new Image of human nature and its applications to education—K-12, as well as Rehabilitative Incarceration.

We acknowledge the similarity of both public, private, and rehabilitative education about the Self as a learning process, which should be available to all humans in all cultures, for the simple reason that if all human cultures use the same accurate image of the species we would likely begin to better understand each other for starters. We have done this in the past unsuccessfully for the reason that we have, almost universally, accepted an ancient image of human nature, based on observational external behavior, based on an impossible set of standards, which was designed to suppress instincts for the control of human behavior. The need of rules for behavioral control existed because it was impossible—and still is impossible—for humans to live up to those standards without open and free use of the natural instincts. This is the center of recent medical and psychological discoveries, and this is the center of the need for a fundamental change in the understanding of learning. We postulate that, if you accept and try to understand the discoveries of psychological and neurological science research of the late 20th century, by the end of the 21st Century your children and grand-children and great grand children will have: "…peace on earth good will toward Men and Women", throughout the world. To reach this realistic goal we will have to place the environments of learning at the top of the agenda of things we must do immediately, and keep it there.

Chapter Eleven. With the age of human nature now validated by the medical research of Dr. Michael Gershon, we are better prepared to fight dis-ease than ever before. It is important that we pay attention to this new consciousness of our two centers of intelligence—two brains—so we can finally make decisions in our lives that care about the whole person, truly reduces stress in our lives, and provides the necessary levels of somatic and psychological nutrients to feed all our needs as human beings. We now can see that we have ignored our humanness, our human nature, and this has led us to great amounts of dis-ease and discomfort. But we live on the cusp of a Renaissance in consciousness of who we truly are and,thus, we can now begin to thrive in this exciting age of our humanity's journey toward a greater life and a more fundamentally intelligent evolution of our species.

Chapter Twelve. In this final chapter, a summary is offered of the cultural and individual importance of following the gut instinctive feelings as a systematic experiential practice that will engender positive states of mind, as well as recapture and utilize the gut response as a dependable center of reference for life decision-making, health and well-being.

*"Once I knew only darkness and stillness... my life was
without past or future... but a little word from the fingers of
another fell into my hand that clutched at emptiness, and my
heart leaped to the rapture of living."*
Helen Keller Preface

INTRODUCTION

This book is a work conceived out of the awareness that directions we take in life often are chosen because of the impact on us of external forces. Judgments of authorities, well-meaning counselors, circumstances, and too often crises dictate the roles we play and the characters we assume, which seldom coincide with our inner needs. Time is wasted day after day and energy is dissipated by each of us pretending that we know what is important while within us is the growing feeling of emptiness.

The experience we have obtained interacting with individuals and groups, provides us with a growing awareness that the feelings, which are ordinarily dealt with, are not pure feeling responses. These so-called feelings are instead, a mixture of thinking and feeling, we commonly call emotions. These logical feelings have a curious universality of meaning, even though these feelings are learned in totally different environments.

Seldom are any of us encouraged to learn to take action as children based on feelings. We seem to grow-up physically, schooled to "think for ourselves" about externalities that are usually only vaguely related to our Selves. If there is any reference in our education and experience to inner necessity, other than food, air, and water, it is carefully molded to conform to patterns of acceptability until only vestiges of human instincts are allowed to show.

And thus we individually live in fear and guilt, angry that we must deny our instinctive feelings and perform in the best way we can, caught between the feeling of need and the judgments of those to whom we want to stay close.

This book was written because of the experience we gained as career counselors trying to reach beneath the surface of many lives of young and old to find what inner needs in them and in ourselves were involved in the emptiness being expressed to us. It was in dealing with the feelings of emptiness that the material in this book was developed. This close contact with persons sponsored reflection on our own lives. Out of this exploration, with others and ourselves, we developed a view of a basic process of decision-making from an inner reference. This view is seen by us as inherent in the process of living, and is clearest when explored by the individual relative to early childhood experiences, usually in the limited environment of the home.

The process of reflection on past experience was developed as a direct result of dealing with emptiness in real life, using inner organismic responses as indicators of the accurate state of awareness of need. While this process of reflection was initiated as a corrective procedure to establish a more positive now, its long term value was found to be in its preventive qualities—its value relating to inner needs in decision-making—so that the person can steer his way through the intricacies of future experience without loosing awareness of his Self, his own state of being. With the use of this dependable inner center, the person can first reference his inner needs and then decide how best to compromise the outer world to satisfy those needs. The process of reflection used in this way—inner needs first—is a way of becoming aware and staying aware of one's Self in the outside world.

The person is seen as caring about and as needing care from all other members of the human race. The common qualities of members of this human race are emphasized and become the common denominators, which support caring and focus attention on the common needs. All of the spatial differences ordinarily used to distinguish us from each other are seen as unimportant details, which tend to separate us and confuse us. With our attention focused on our differences, we establish artificial barriers that prevent caring and communicating our needs. To us, the human race is seen as a family of persons needing to get close to each other, and learning about themselves from each other by finding themselves in each other.

We would like to thank the Sonoma State University Psychology Department for its support in offering an educational environment in which recent research using the Somatic Reflection Process was conducted. We give particular thanks to Dr. Laurel McCabe, Dr. Susan Stewart, Reverend Dr. Jeremy Taylor, Dr. Geri Olson, Dr. Greg Bogart, Dr. David Sowerby and Maureen Murdock, M.F.T. for their teaching capacity and writing assistance on the original material on the Somatic Reflection Process submitted as a thesis in 2005. We would also like to thank Dr. Eleanor Criswell Hanna for both supporting our publication of material in Somatics Magazine and allowing us the freedom to reprint sections of those articles in this book.

Also, we thank all those who have throughout the last 40 years participated with us in exploring the Somatic Reflection Process in coaching sessions as well as in our research efforts. Even though you are too numerous to name, we will always remember you.

"We do not remember days, we remember moments."
Cesare Pavese

CHAPTER ONE:

DEVELOPMENT OF THE CONCEPT OF REFLECTION ON GUT INSTINCTS

The following is a summary of the development of the process of reflecting on the basic inner somatic gut feelings, which is directed toward achieving a higher awareness of the inner Self. We developed this process through interaction with hundreds of individuals as well as with individuals in groups in a community college. The community college setting provided us with the opportunity to interact with each other around this experience and thus allowed us to experience a higher Self-awareness along with our clients and students. The result is that we were able to explore in our-Selves the depth of awareness that comes from the use of the inner somatic feelings in reflection and discover the methodology for this reflection process.

To suggest that a somatic inner instinctive accountability exists with a reliable and constant organismic rationale or intelligence, which must be served by the logical thinking process in order to maintain a state of health, may be seen as an unseemly contradiction of tradition—and it is. Such a concept, however does find its way into view through the simple respect for the feeling judgment when learned patterns of external, logical, systems of thought are bypassed. When experience is examined in retrospect from the point of view of "what the organism needed in prospect," it is possible to discover what we call the "impact of experience"—the inner value of the experience to the organism. This approach to human experience reveals a universality of purpose, which we have begun to identify as "instinctive need" as it seems to be the same in all human beings. Differences, which the phenomenologists describe, seem to be the result of learning a coping-style in order for the organism to try to satisfy its binary instinctive needs in relation to its environments.

The following discussion is an account of the experiential path we have followed in individual and group work, which has brought us to our concept of the nature and use of instincts in human experience. The initial purpose of our work was to counsel students and persons in the community college about choices of careers and the educational routes to take toward those choices. All clients were voluntary, as was the use of the Myers-Briggs Type Indicator (MBTI), which provided personality data to suggest a learning and coping style in support of career choice possibilities. We will be discussing the MBTI at length in a later chapter.

Early experience indicated (primarily from the MBTI results) that it was often unclear for whom the occupational choice was being made. Often choices were directed by fathers, mothers, friends or relatives, which had no relationship to the persons coping style nor feeling about himself or herself.

Persons from the community looking for retraining or a change in career, upon reflection on past careers, could validate two aspects in their experience: (1) It was not the knowledge or the training they had that determined their success or failure in their work but their ability to cope with the work environment—their feeling about themselves in relation to the dynamics of the environment of things and persons, and (2) With the MBTI results, they could realize that the difference that existed between their coping style and what was required of them in the type of work they had been doing, had resulted in negative feelings about their experience, as well as negative feelings quite often about themselves.

Our classroom experience as counselors in self-awareness groups, provided us with a growing awareness that the feelings expressed by people, with which we were dealing in class with the Myers-Briggs Type Indicator (MBTI) results, were a mixture of thinking and feeling—a consideration by the logical brain about the details of an experience that was psychological in nature, along with a feeling that was a body gut response about the same experience and somatic in nature—that was combined together in what may be called psycho-somatic feelings.

The psychosomatic thinking-feeling responses had a curious universality of meaning even though they were learned in totally different environments by many people. Such feelings as guilt, fear, and hostility seemed to be clearly understood even though no one had ever taken a formal lesson in either one. When anyone in our class groups would express a feeling of guilt, everyone knew what was meant. The same was true for fear—the feeling was universally understood. No one ever seemed to misunderstand the person who was expressing hostility. These names indicated a common response in all individuals and set us on a curious course to discover more about this universality.

The MBTI served as an explicit model of the personality or coping style, which allowed for a more positive assessment of the phenomenological Self—the external self that makes up our individual personality. With its use, a person could view themselves with less guilt when they could see their experience in terms of this MBTI model. Often people found they had blamed themselves for difficulties that were resulted simply from a difference in personality styles with other key people in their lives. The reduced guilt for being oneself rather than focusing on the details for which one felt the guilt, made people feel less odd about themselves and more interested in reassessing past experience in terms of this model—this new understanding of oneself.

We became aware that it was important to perfect the process of reflection in order to deal effectively with guilt. It is interesting in retrospect to realize that the feeling judgment seen in the MBTI model, and the guilt being dealt with by people in their present lives has a past time frame of reference, which was stored at the time of experience and accessible upon reflection on the past. The Myers-Briggs directed us toward a feeling of acceptability in a phenomenological sense. We realized that, when we felt acceptable in a phenomenal sense, we might approach total acceptance of our selves in the present. Our first efforts in reflecting were around guilt, fear and hostility using the Myers-Briggs as a structure for Self-Awareness. But this experience seemed to point to similarities in feelings, which were not covered by the differences described in the various MBTI coping styles. It did not take long to become aware that these named feelings were derived from a common response center and are named from the contextual aspects of the experience. That is, all seemed to be the same feeling separated by the logical context in which they were named. One of these elements in the context was clearly a matter of time—past, present, and future, and the other was clearly a matter of space—people, places and thing around us.

We experienced the logical "negative" feelings—guilt, fear, and hostility—as positive signs indicating an organismic need, without which there would be no conscious awareness of any unfilled inner needs. We became aware that beneath these logical feelings there was a gut response, which simply registered empty or full when we were aware of these logical feelings. When we got to the gut' feelings, we found that by sharing these responses early at a low level of intensity, we could reduce the feelings of guilt, fear, and hostility. By reflecting on these gut feelings, we could find a more fundamental organismic issue, which was triggered in by the contextual phenomenal feelings. We began to realize that we experienced an infinite number of logical feelings—joy, sorrow, doubt, love, hate, etc.—all of which relate to a simple binary response of empty-full in the gut region of the organism.

We then turned our attention to the gut feelings in reflection and began to see that the gut was responding to basic, simple needs of the organism. When guilt was being expressed in a situational context and we asked the person the source of the guilt, he would point to situational details as the cause. His logic would select the phenomenological possibility of his feelings. With a little care—time and attention—a more fundamental emptiness, a gut response would ultimately come into awareness, which we began to view as a form of the feeling of acceptance. By chasing this feeling concerned with acceptance back through time and experience, concentrating on the basic feeling, we would consistently end up around the ages of 3, 4, or 5 years of age in some close relationship when this first feeling of lack of acceptance was high in the childhood awareness. In all of the reflective situations the details changed, yet the impact remained consistent. It was not until an organismic purpose could be felt by the reflector that a lessening of guilt was experienced.

When fear was expressed by a person in the present, upon reflection into the past the feeling of guilt would immediately take its place. Only when we would concentrate on futuristic possibilities would fear be a logical feeling priority. Operating from an organismic gut feeling of emptiness in the now, we found guilt associated with past details, fear associated with future details of expectation, and hostility as an expression of feeling 'trapped' in the logical now. Dealing with the future possibilities from the now gut response, the person would ultimately describe a basic feeling of being "out of control" in relation to the future. No relief was experienced until a fuller feeling in the now could be experienced, which in turn was reflected as less guilt about acceptance in the past and again, in turn, as a brighter prospect of being in control of the future.

This pattern of acceptance and control became such a consistent pattern of our experience in class groups and with individual clients, that we cautiously and tentatively labeled them 'instinctive' responses. We could see that we were reflecting on inner qualities—Self-Acceptance and Self-Control—but the extension of the concept could be expanded to outer qualities—acceptance by others and control of others. We thus could tie the inner somatic response of emptiness to awareness of the lack of inner organismic needs satisfaction and to MBTI feelings and external patterns of behavior. While the MBTI coping style was highlighting differences between persons, our newfound awareness of organismic feelings pointed to the consistency and sameness in all human experience.

We then began to take Kant's time and space a priori elements of experience seriously. Time became a factor of perception and judgment—sensing, now time; intuition, future time; feeling, past time; and thinking (logic) covered all three time frames as a bonding process. Guilt, fear, and hostility curiously had logical time frames in coincidence with Jung's processes of sensing, intuiting, and feeling. The coping styles—Jung's personality types—provided a time awareness, which tied the inner awareness , our gut feelings, to the outer awareness of the phenomenological feelings. It was as a result of this discovery that the meaning of experience—the impact of experience—is seen as a qualitative use of time, which becomes an inner experience in contrast with the outer awareness of space.

Space was understood as that aspect of experience that is derived from sense data (sight, sound, taste, touch, and smell). These senses are seen as externally oriented to provide information on the state of space in the individual's present environment. A space has expansive dimensions, qualities, which time does not, and the senses, in a priority system, provide data for both the thinking and feeling, which the organism uses if response—immediate action—is required. The logical feelings to which we refer are the result of this combined thinking/feeling judgment. Our concern with the MBTI adaptation of Carl Jung's personality types was that it does not allow for the deeper inner somatic feeling response (in the body), therefore, it fails to adequately discriminate between logic and feeling. It seems to obtain this logic/feeling mixture of phenomenological experience and it does not sufficiently separate logic and feeling. We have presently abandoned the use of the MBTI for the reasons that it points to phenomenological differences in coping and does not provide for the experience of pure logic and pure somatic feelings. Feelings are considered in the MBTI structure, as did Jung, as judgments of value, but this judgment is not pure somatic feeling nor described in somatic terms. Without such qualities of separation of thinking and feeling, the logic could never be distracted by outside authorities or be taught—educated to accept external systems of thought such as abstractions like ethics, theology, good, bad, etc. Without such separation, the feelings could not represent the basic nature of organism—there would not be a conflict between two rational centers; thinking—"I should"—"I should not", and feeling—the fact that " I feel 'empty' or I feel 'full'.

One of our early attractions to the idea that the human being operates around inner instinctive necessities of quite primitive somatic origin was that whatever these basic issues are, they must be available prior to complex thinking awareness at birth. It was also clear to us that they must have been available to the species in some early primitive pre-verbal state. In other words, they must be consistent and constant to mark the species and not a learned variable.

We learned through the process of reflection on somatic feeling responses that, beginning in early childhood, the issues of acceptance and control are active principles; that childhood is an active experimental period around these issues; and that while not specially mobile, the child is in control of his responses in his environment, covertly and overtly as required, toward gaining acceptance by those close to him. The experimental effort at this time before school is directed toward developing a coping style—a copy at first—to deal with the control and acceptance issues. When we reflected chronologically up through time we found these preschool patterns recycling and compounding in new experience still dealing with the same issues, desperately trying to strike a balance between them—exploring out into the person's perceptual field but always checking for acceptance of his and her new experience with him or herself. This we found to be a totally inner process, which external behavior would not reliably reveal. Behavior, often pointed away from the person's feelings when he or she had learned the necessity to hide them. The person's behavior was a highly deceptive screen if he or she had learned in early experience that outer judgments reflected unacceptability of his and her inner feelings. The person's feelings were clear to him or herself and were clearly registered as a record of that time and were available, upon reflection on those issues, to him or her and to communicate to others who care about how he or she felt then. This becomes the record of the person's life with no loss of important information when he or she can be encouraged by being given the time and attention to reflect at that basic level of organismic purpose.

When we could see the universality of the issues of Acceptance and Control, in hundreds of persons both young and old, we could see these issues as so basic to the human species that we felt confident that they were responses at an organismic level and identified them as the human instincts.

THE PURPOSE:
REASSESSING THE MEANING OF EXPERIENCE

The meaning of the present and the future depends upon the meaning of past experience. In order to be clearly aware of the distinction between external systems of thought and instinctive feeling responses, it is helpful to reflect on instinctive feelings of fullness and emptiness at times when the concept of the experience was simple—on times when responses were more instinctive and less influenced by external authority. In this way is it possible to assess the impact on the organism of past experience, free the perception to deal in the now, and set the positive expectation for the future.

If in a person's reflection, the impact of experience is lacking in awareness, then the meaning of experience is derived from logical external observed details in relation to external systems of thought. Such an assessment may be applied in the now, either from judgments applied in the now coming in directly from the present environment or one the person automatically applies from judgments experienced out of the past, and thus the future prospect of experience contains the expectation of the same situational judgment. Meaning of one's past experience is subject to evaluation by the inner necessity of the organism and also to the acceptance of the external system of logical thought.

The prospect of experience is always based upon inner feeling and derives necessity from perceived instinctive needs. There may be an awareness of logical positions against such a prospect but the driving force is inner feeling regardless of the developed rationale for outside deception. The organism drives toward inner fullness and away from emptiness in its attempt to balance control of its responses and acceptance of those responses in experience. After the fact of experience, when a reflection on the meaning begins, a shift from the inner objective to an external logical objective often occurs.

The shift to logical thought assessment occurs because there has been a happening and the evidence is often in full view of others. At this point inner prospect becomes outer retrospect and demands a logical rationale. The external logical rationale often omits the inner prospect, which was never explicit because of its questioned acceptability by the controlling organism. Control was taken in prospect often with questioned acceptability but in retrospect, with the evidence in full view, there is little choice but to submit to the external judgments relative to the acceptability of the results and to forget what purpose to the organism was intended. Such confusion in the assessment of experience constitutes a loss of purpose to the person and an empty prospect for future openness.

The reflection on instinctive feelings as a process is an attempt to get at the original objective—what the person was trying to accomplish for itself—without applying the external judgment it encountered in retrospect to the original experience. It is a reassessment of experience in favor of instinctive necessity at the time the prospective point of view was determined.

Since the retrospective view is observed external to the organism and is concerned with some external system of logical thought; religious, social, economic, ethics or morality, the judgments are concerned with the details of the happening rather than a purposeful objective in the satisfaction of the inner needs of the organism. Such judgments—prior to the logical, rational, maturity, the organism—are taken by the person as against his inner instinctive nature. He is likely to experience a rejection of his inner nature and hide his instinctive feelings from others, when possible. He will learn to gain control in devious ways and try to gain acceptance, often with bizarre behavior as a result.

Reflection on the impact of experience, which reopens experience to the organism's purposeful instinctive objectives, is an attempt to reestablish the credibility of instinctive needs, increase sensitivity to instinctive gut feelings and let the organism begin to trust its natural instinctive responses as in early childhood. As awareness to these natural feelings is gained and their reliability in coping with the world of people and things is reestablished, there is greater reliance on internal authority and less need for external authority. Through such awareness a more caring person emerges, creative productivity increases, and more constructive energy is available for maintenance of a healthy organism.

SPONTANEOUS SHARING OF INSTINCTIVE FEELINGS: THE MEANINGFUL USE OF TIME

A higher awareness of somatic instinctive feelings developed by the reflection process on feelings, not only provides a reassessment of past experience, but it also provides an openness to the expression of basic feelings, and also provides an invitation for others to communicate their feelings. This sharing of feelings provides accuracy in a relationship for caring for each other since it discloses the instinctive needs of each person in a relationship from moment to moment. The elimination of guesswork in a human relationship makes it possible to see the sameness in each other and minimizes the coping stylistic differences, which are all too easily perceived from the outside. The experience of sharing of instinctive feelings in all situations allows persons to experience closeness and understanding and eliminates the need for guilt in retrospect and eliminates fear of the next prospect. Such experience in a relationship reduces the use of wasted maintenance energy on unresolved issues stemming from guilt. It guides the energy toward constructive qualities in the relationship and reduces the need for uncontrolled bursts of energy in a seemingly destructive use of hostility. With a higher awareness of the basic issues in a relationship derived from knowing the feelings of another person, the time spent with them has a greater and rewarding value. It provides for the most meaningful use of time.

The reflection on instinctive common human feeling responses stresses a vital role for the logical thinking process. The logic seems to have been designed for use by each organism but is early in our development distracted to use by external authorities. The weakness of logic is that the premise from which conclusions are drawn may or may not be relevant to the needs of the organism. If the premise of the human thinking-logical process is irrelevant to the organisms needs, the conclusions derived from that premise will also be irrelevant. If, however, the premise is based on the instinctive needs of the person, then the conclusions of logical needs satisfaction will be directed toward that end—the needs of the organism.

With awareness of its needs and the use of its logic system to direct it toward those needs—a balance between control and acceptance of its responses in time and space—the organism can take full responsibility for its feelings and begin to drop the need to pretend, to play roles, and to project the blame for its feelings on external situations or other persons. The inability of each of us to say a decisive "yes" or "no" to external situations or persons instead of "maybe" is a common dilemma. If we can know the "pay-off" to the Self by being sensitive to the empty-full feelings our gut provides, instead of the "should" and "should-not" of external systems of thought, we may well experience our Selves and others in a way that sweeps away guilt from the past, that provides meaningful use of time in the now and avoids fear of what is to come in the future— a major daily reduction of stress.

"Only those who will risk going too far can possibly find out how far one can go."
T. S. Eliot

CHAPTER TWO:

MEDICAL BREAKTHROUGH SUPPORTS THE GUT AS A CENTER OF INTELLIGENCE

Recent neurological discoveries of the nature of human intelligence inform us of new images of the human nervous systems. The new image is of two nervous systems, one connected to the upper brain, and another, neurological research has found, connected to the ancient 'snake brain'. Each brain controls its own nervous system independent of the other, yet they can communicate with each other, and coordinate their separate functions to support the human organism to function as a single unit. The significance of the discovery is that the image now includes two centers of intelligence instead of just one. The presence of two centers of intelligence provides the organism with the answers to some of the inner mysteries over which man has pondered for centuries.

This image includes the primary focus of the upper brain, with its sensory awareness of the organism's external environment, and of *the second brain* (Gershon, 1998) or gut brain, with its primary focus on the organism's inner needs satisfaction, providing a somatic feeling awareness of the organism's energy production, and managing the entire electrochemical feeling responses of the human digestive system. The feeling responses of the digestive system seems to be closely related to the well-being of the organism.

When cognitive awareness is combined with the inner feeling experience of human needs satisfaction, a person seems to be using more of the natural talents available to cope with life. The experience of the inner feeling of needs satisfaction seems to require a special focus on inner body awareness in order to balance body needs with the overwhelming sensory input. This sensory information is often counter-productive to living a mentally and physically healthy life. By focusing more on the inner feeling awareness, the impact of experience and what the experience means to a person, a better balance of important information to the person's needs seems to be achieved. These two separate nervous systems, when operating in concert, are available to guide the human organism toward fulfilling its design objectives. The unique, individual design objectives are formulated at conception as the architecture of the person to be, and these design objectives remain active throughout the entire life.

In order to reach the inner feeling awareness, it seems necessary to be sensitive to the feelings of the internal body responses, past and present, along with the cognitive responses, past and present, to the outside environment. The past seems to be stored for future reference in both the upper brain and the body. The body, therefore, must have a mind of its own—the actual result of the neurological research of Dr. Michael Gershon. We postulate, as a result of recent medical research and our clinical experience, that we were dealing with a quality of intelligence, common and available to all human beings. It is our hope in this book to identify images that will help people achieve awareness and balance between these two centers of intelligence—mind and belly.

Our clinical work in the 1970s was done mainly with post high school students who could not meet the college academic entrance standards of the time, or were back from Viet Nam and were looking for an occupation, or were foreign students working on college entrance requirements, or were trying desperately to come back from drug related addictions. Nearly all of them needed personal counseling and expressed stress symptoms of confusion and anxiety, often with difficulties sleeping, finding adequate energy to function at work or school, or maintaining satisfying personal relationships.

Counseling using the Somatic Reflection Process (SRP) was an unproven, unpublished theory in the 1970s. We, who used SRP in Behavioral Science Classes, in groups, and with individuals, found very little interest among the faculty where we worked. The encouragement we received was from the students who participated in this method of attention. When we wrote the text: *Borne Of the Human Family* for our classes in 1975, we were convinced that there was something special going on in the gut area that gave access to much more useful information to the counselee than anything taught in the profession at that time. It was in 1998 that Dr. Gershon published his research results that offered a credible explanation for the gut response with which we had been working.

THE WORLD OF THE ENTERIC NERVOUS SYSTEM

The most significant discovery relative to education has been in the field of neurobiology. The scientific research, begun in 1958 by a young student at Cornel University, who was fascinated with the ability of LSD to block the affects of the chemical Serotonin on organs of the rat. At that time, LSD was a highly experimental drug, and serotonin, known to be present in the brain, was thought, to be involved in the mind-altering effects of LSD. Since the brain looked too complicated to the young man, and the effect of LSD on a rat organ was associated with the lower body, the student chose the body for what he thought would be an easier study. As it turned out, Dr. Michael Gershon, who is now generally known as the father of modern neurogastroenterology, became involved in a systematic discovery of the nature of the nervous system that controlled the human bowel. After thirty years of work he describes the detailed struggle with his research and the disbelief of his peers, in his book, *The Second Brain: Your Gut Has a Mind of It's Own*. This book is not only a major advancement in the field of medicine, the digestive system, but it provides a clear image and the function of the organs of the human digestive tract as they relate to the mental processes of the main brain. And it is only this main brain that we as educators have tried to influence since public education was invented. The image we educators have used, and still apply, consists of the main brain and the heart. The main brain turns out to involve less than half of the intellectual capacity of the human organism, and the heart is one of the organs influenced by this newly discovered enteric nervous system, along with the stomach, the liver, the gall bladder, the pancreas, the large intestine, the small intestine, the anus, and all of the valves and mussels that regulate the electro-chemical, digestive processes from the throat to the anus. Perhaps the upper brain and the heart have been given credit for intelligence that the gut deserved.

If we can think in terms of energy for a moment, the food in the digestive tract is the energy source, the fuel for the generator providing the energy used throughout the body. The enteric nervous system influences the distribution network that circulates that energy to every part of the body, even the upper brain. These two vital functions are at the center of the organism that keep the system ticking regardless of what the upper brain is dealing. On the other hand what the main upper brain is thinking affects the gut. The sensory data from the upper brain is either in support of or in conflict with the energy source, the operation of the enteric nervous system. We have all felt reactions in the gut from that with which the mind is dealing. Tightness, a physical feeling when a conflict exists between the two systems, and relaxation, a physical feeling when the conflict is resolved. The expectation and resolution is a condition commonly called, "butterflies in the stomach". If more serious problems exist, we can experience feelings in the stomach of cramps, diarrhea, constipation, and vomiting and all of these body feelings are forms of intelligent control of the body process by the enteric nervous system. In general, every tissue within the body cavity is connected and influenced by the enteric nervous system, and every tissue outside the body cavity is connected and controlled by the central nervous system. This division of labor makes sense when the body functions are carefully examined.

The central nervous system functions primarily as a sensory receiver and manager of outside information and outside activity for the organism. The enteric nervous system functions primarily as the source and manager of energy production, as we pointed out before. These two systems are intimately connected together to operate the human organism, to maintain and inform each other of what is going on in real time, and to maintain an accurate historical record of each function throughout life. The upper brain, with the central nervous system, records the images it constructs from sensory data it experiences over time. The gut, with the enteric nervous system, records the impact of the same experiences over time, but with an accurate measure of the value—threat to or strength for— the entire organism with a positive or negative feeling.

A short distance beyond the teeth and stretching for yards of wrinkled flexible tubing, sized to fit varying physical requirements, lays the complicated electrochemical domain of the enteric nervous system. Its design seems to be to use this tubular contraption to provide energy for whatever an unseen demand calls—something like a signal from the Captain on the bridge to the engine room in the lowest part of a ship. Like the ship, the enteric nervous system (ENS) is equipped with a communications system that allows it to manage the "engine room" and simultaneously communicate with the Captain who is steering the ship with the sensory information from what he senses is going on outside.

This functional separation of two vital needs of the ship and the organism seems to provide for immediate action when quick moves and energy are necessary for such a move to be available on demand. This bilateral communication also allows for the sensory data (sight, sound, taste, touch, and smell) to be received and logged (stored) by the central nervous system (CNS) and the impact data, the internal, operational data to be logged in the ENS. The logging of the data of the two systems provides information for planning (thinking) between the two systems to better prepare (intuition) for the future possibilities.

CONCLUSIONS ON GERSHON'S RESEARCH

We have tried to capture the essence of Dr. Gershon's research without pretending to know the intricacies of the each organ that is operationally managed by the ENS. The use of the analogue is only one of many human developments that have used the human anatomy as a developmental model. Whether this developmental phenomenon is conscious or unconscious, we can't say, but we have yet to find a single man-made system that does not reflect some form of the human system—even adaptability. We have also learned to distort these natural qualities of control and acceptance to gain power over each other. The natural qualities will be more evident when we look closely at the development of the fetus.

This conclusion gives us pause to wonder why we have so much trust in the dependability of the human model when we relate to things, and so much distrust in our human nature when we apply the model to human social issues? We could be using the dependability of the human anatomy as an analogue for ethics and morality instead of an analogue for depravation.

THE WORLD OF THE FETUS FOUND TO BEGIN IN THE GUT

We offer another breakthrough of research and theory in neuroscience by Dr. Lise Eliot as relevant to the validation of our clinical work on the instinctual gut response. It seems to us that the body intelligence, which is in charge of the development and repair process for the life of the organism, resides in the original or the differentiated form of every cell in the body. If this idea is correct, then a closer look at what has and does go on in the human organism from conception to maturity is important. This information should give us some idea of our role as educators and parents in the development of each child as a unique organism. With a better understanding of the characteristics of the individual student, we can fashion an educational program to enhance the outcome, and provide the individual child with a more conscious awareness of his potential. Then, we can provide him the tools to reach his potential centered on his individual needs.

Beginning at conception, potential is provided to the future organism by the parents as the master plan, the DNA (the architectural plan) and the RNA (the contractor that builds the system), metaphorically speaking. Unless some outside force distorts this program, this DNA/RNA combination will remain with the organism throughout its life. The building process is designed to follow a specific time schedule with specific parts of the organism provided in a specific order, very much as any man-made structure would be built. Therefore, a timeline of the process is designed for the completion of each critical phase of the construction, in order for the next phase to begin. Like any building process, some aspects of the construction take place in parallel with others as long as the objective of the critical phase is met.

FETAL CONSTRUCTION SCHEDULE: FERTILIZATION TO BIRTH—9 MONTHS

The following simplistic chart was organized from information we have taken from a book by neuroscientist Dr. Lise Eliot, Ph.D. (1999) titled *What's Going On In There: How the Brain and Mind Develop in the First Five Years of Life*:

First Month	Zygote attaches to lining of uterus / rapid cell division / beginning of enteric (digestive) nervous system.
Second Month	Heart and blood vessels form / head area develops / arm and leg stubs form / sex shows / digestive system and internal organs show / heart beats faintly. Embryo: 1" long / weight 1/10oz.
Third Month	Digestive system begins functioning / bones begin to grow / vestigial limbs show

	movement. Fetus: 3"long / weight 1oz.
Fourth Month	Detectable heart beat/bones seen by x-ray / lower body parts grow rapidly.
	Fetus: 5"long / weight 5oz.
Fifth Month	Ears and nose show cartilage / fingers and toes show nails/ hiccups/ thumb
	Sucking / kicking in evidence / body covered with waxy-fuzz (Vernix) coating.
	Fetus: 7" long / weight 14oz.
Sixth Month	Fat develops under skin / eyes fully developed.
	Fetus: 11-14" long / weight 1-1/2lbs.
Seventh Month	Cerebral brain develops rapidly.
	Fetus: 15-16"long / weight 3lbs.
Eighth Month	Fat is stored / nails extending.
	Fetus: 17" long / weight 5lbs.
Ninth Month	Final development: testing enteric nervous system in preparation for birth / body covering is shed / baby assumes head-down position to enter the birth canal / birth occurs when the baby signals it's ready to function outside the womb.
	Baby: Roughly 21" long / weight 7lbs.

It may seem, initially, that the treatment of the development of the fetus and the metaphor we have used as a building process is an imaginative distortion, and it may be. But the reason why we have used it is because it is a paradigm for what we are about to present. If we can stand back and look at what is revealed by the reproductive process, we think we can present an argument for the meaning of this process to possibly all of man's discoveries—the fruits of his intuition, imagination; and serve as a paradigm that supports his sensory achievements. Man is not a creator; he copies what nature reveals to him—consciously or unconsciously.

CONCLUSIONS ON FETAL DEVELOPMENT

Looking at the first three months of fetal development, it seems clear that the first complete aspect of the organism is its digestive system. The digestive system is established and is operating, without help from any other completed internal system, between the third and fourth month of gestation. No upper brain is there to direct its function. No source of instruction except the original DNA/RNA exists. All of the intelligence that is available is in the Master Plan, the DNA. And all of the intelligence available to the builder is in the RNA, and all of the building materials to be used in the construction are manufactured on site.

The almost infinite variety of different cells, used throughout construction are differentiated (formed) from stem cells at the construction site, (assembly yard) and directed to where the final organs or tissues will ultimately reside in the structure. The undifferentiated stem cells continue to divide when materials for repair jobs are needed after the original plan is finished. This image seems to us to be one of a universal intelligence that sets in motion the destiny of all life. This inner intelligence will be of a size and complexity to meet the master plan and needs of the organism, and we need to be cognizant of it and consciously engage it.

It is by going down into the abyss that we recover the
treasures of life. Where you stumble, there lies your treasure.

Joseph Campbell

CHAPTER THREE:

THE IMPACT OF EXPERIENCE:

THE UNIVERSAL PRINCIPLES
OF FEELINGS

Today is felt to be the most complicated day in our lives and rarely in trying to deal with the issues of today, are we aware of the impact of the past on those issues. As we try to sort through the details of what is going on around us, we are often unable to see a clear positive path into the future. It seems no matter what we do to take action on the issues the same empty feeling persists or reoccurs and the actions seem only to further complicate the issue, leaving the emptiness to be dealt with later on.

It seems to be quite natural for us to try to figure out what is bothering us—to understand what is going on. Usually, as long as we keep the reflection to ourselves, we continually see the details and fail to find the meaning of the issue. Even though we reach out to a friend and ask for attention around the details of the issue, we may gain little or no insight into what is bothering us. Often the attention we get is sympathy for having to deal with the details of the issue. We become quite confused about ourselves and we get hostile at the one to whom we have asked for help and have gotten sympathy. Such an experience with another person focusing on details, serves only to leave us feeling more empty and alone.

As we comb through the piles of details of the past, we know in our feelings that the details weren't the meaning of the experience. Somehow through the external judgments we used in the assessment of the experience, we become too confused to understand this clearly. As a child, we often move into action with our instinctive feelings, often with no logical motive. Others who observe our actions are privy only to the details and often make judgments about us from what they can perceive, without an understanding of our feelings.

If we enter experience from our instinctive feelings, we must assess the meaning of the experience from the original feeling needs involved. We must exclude other external logical judgments if we wish to understand clearly what our behavior means. Only by such a reflective process—reflection with the inner gut feelings—is the confusion eliminated.

When we can push the details of the experience out of our awareness, we can turn into the awareness of ourselves and reflect on our inner feelings. It is when we can do this that we are able to see the relationship of the confusion of the present to the issues and the feelings of the past. It is only through the process of reflection on our feelings, triggered in the confusion of the present, that we can begin to understand the sources of the feelings that are causing the confusion. By dealing with these past feelings, we may begin to arrive at some understanding with what we are dealing in the present moment.

These feelings accumulated from our past, rather than the details of our lives, seem to be the accurate record of the impact of our life experience. Until we perceive these early childhood feelings as acceptable, the patterns that develop with time constantly interfere with our understanding of ourselves in the past. Not until these feelings are validated by another person as acceptable human feelings can we let go of the past and put our full energies into present experience.

Fear, guilt, hostility—with an underlying emptiness feeling—triggered in by our present experiences are signals telling us that there is a need to reflect upon the past issues up through time in order to free ourselves from the past unresolved feelings about ourselves. The surface logical feelings of guilt and fear signal to us a conflict between what we think and what we feel about ourselves. A conflict or lack of communication is going on between our gut feelings and logical thinking brain. On the basis of our feeling awareness, the reflection up through time shows us the necessity for the actions we have taken.

The instinctive feeling of emptiness is signaling our logical mind that there is unfinished work to be done. There is an inner and outer conflict to be resolved and a reckoning of our two brains, the beginning of which lies festering in our past experiences. Once we find the source of the original disturbance, in the often distant past, reflecting back through time identifying the occasions when the feelings of emptiness matched the feeling of the now—the same feeling and likely reoccurring at several different ages; we need to clarify the purpose we were trying to achieve by the action and what need we were trying to fill. Then we need to work our way back in time in reflection touching the same occasions of emptiness we found before, and clarifying each instance all the way up to the present. It is then that we have become aware of much about ourselves and our environments, which we have been unaware before, and now we can realize the necessity of dealing with experience from our inner center of intelligence as well as the outer sensory judgment of others.

A PROCESS OF SELF-AWARENESS

The best way to understand how the impact of experiences in the present trigger us to respond from our feelings that are related to unresolved issues in the past, is to go through the process yourself around an issue you are struggling with in the present time. We often ask our clients in counseling to describe in their feelings the impact of the issue they are struggling with. And if it isn't clear to them what we were talking about, we ask them to find in their own mind and feelings something about their life that if they could resolve would help make life much better. We ask them not to tell us the details but try to describe the feeling in their body. Then we begin the process of taking the feelings they are having and reflecting on their feelings back to an earlier time in their past when they had that feeling before, as young as possible. It is through this Somatic Reflection Process (SRP) that original issues become conscious, sometimes for the first time since they happened, and people can work through them to change their self-image, and find understanding to resolve the present issues.

In the following example of the Somatic Reflection Process[1], the person was faced in the present issue with fulfilling unsuitable demands from others as a requirement for continued employment and this required choices between doing what felt necessary for this person and doing what authorities at work expected. As the reflection process proceeds, the feeling of this present situation reminds this person of similar choices made all the way back to childhood. While this problem concerns a career choice in the present, it sponsors feelings that deal with the major unresolved issues in the person's life including sexuality, which might ordinarily seem unrelated to a career choice.

54

Facilitator (F): Could you look at the most unresolved issue in your life and center on the feelings?

Reflector(R): When I see somebody needing or hurting for something that I can furnish, and if I don't feel like furnishing it, then I feel guilty for not doing it.

F: You think you're going to loose something by doing?

R: If I do something because someone expects me to—yeah—I lose something—I end up empty.

F: When you think you should pour yourself into someone else?

R: I do something for them—I think I should—because they seem empty and then I end up empty.

F: Can you find a face connected with this present feeling and look carefully back into the past to find a time when you felt this feeling before?

R: You mean a face I relate this feeling to now?

F: Yes, right now.

R: OK—I've found a face. An important one.

F: Does this seem to be an important issue in your feelings?

R: Yes, it's probably the most important unresolved issue. One that I would like to work out.

F: Is there only one face connected with this feeling?

R: No. I think I can connect this feeling with nearly everyone I know.

F: Can you find a time in your life in the past when you felt this way before? Try to go back.

R: Should I trace it back? Do you mean—yeah, I find it at about 16.

F: Would you restate the feeling as you look at the faces around you at that time?

R: I feel like I would not be acceptable to people, if I didn't do things for them that they said they needed.

F: Whose faces are important in that?

R: Friends!

F: Anyone else?

R: My parents?

F: Which faces are the most important to you at that time?

R: I seem to be caught between them all.

F: You feel you are pulled in several directions?

R: I'm not sure any of those directions are for me.

F: Are you centered on a particular experience?

R: It seems that it occurred over and over again. Like, if I wasn't going to be alone, I would have to consider other people's feelings first before mine no matter how I felt about it. I would feel guilty if I didn't do that, and if I did, hostile for doing that when I didn't feel like it. And no one seemed to care. Guilty that I felt that way—that maybe I was odd.

F: You should be glad to furnish their needs?

R: There might be something sexually wrong with me. I was always expected to "give out". That was a very common feeling.

F: Maybe you can find that same feeling earlier— probably around other details in your life?

R: The feeling that I should do something for someone else that I didn't want to do. That I would be unacceptable and alone if I didn't?

F: Yes. Can you find that same feeling in an earlier time?

R: Earlier? Let's see—yes. I felt that way when I was eight or nine.

F: What was the feeling at eight?

R: Hostility. I felt controlled because I couldn't show how I really felt.

F: Whose faces are associated with it at the time?

R: My aunt—my mother and father—their faces come in pretty strong. The clearest feeling that is the same as the one we started with is going to auntie's house and here she comes after me. Standing there at the door having to pretend I liked it when she would kiss me on the mouth.

F: What was the feeling?

R: The guilt that I resented her for that, and the hostility for not being able to show my feeling about her.

F: That sounds very much like the original feeling, doesn't it?

R: Maybe we need to look at that closer because that happened over and over. That's the only clear feeling I can remember early—seemed like that happened all my life.

F: How long did this go on?

R: Until she died.

F: Can you get a specific time in your mind and focus on your feelings around the details?

R: OK! I'm back there, I think like four or five years old. It felt like—she was coming to kiss me—I had to smile and physically respond on the outside without showing hostility. I had to let her do whatever she wanted to do to me and pretend that I liked it

F: What was the feeling?

R: Angry! I felt like no one cared how I felt. My feelings were not acceptable. I felt alone and empty.

F: Can you look at the other faces in your feelings around that scene?

R: Mother seems to be important.

F: What is the feeling in relation to her?

R: Guilt if I didn't perform.

F: It was her judgment that you should perform?

R: Yes, I thought that if I didn't I would hurt her—I thought she would be unacceptable to my father. It seemed to me at that time that all of us—me, my sisters, and my mother, would be unacceptable to my father if we didn't perform and show my aunt that we loved her.

F: How do you feel as you see his face?

R: Guilty—if he knew how hostile I felt about my aunt—his sister. I was afraid I wouldn't be acceptable. He was gone away a lot and I was afraid he might go away and I'd feel alone. You know, now that I feel through that time, it seemed in my feelings that he left because of the problems we all caused him. But, I can see now that it was his work—but as a young child—I didn't know what the word "work" meant and thought he was leaving because of me. I think I decided that hostility was destructive and it made people go away from each other. I can see now that he may not really have wanted to go because if his feelings about me—but to take care of the family, to work.

F: Now come back up to a more recent experience with those feelings of guilt and hostility.

R: Yeah! I never would just tell someone how hostile I felt toward them—I was afraid that would make them go away.

F: Where does the guilt come from?

R: The guilt was that I should perform even though that wasn't what I needed—I felt guilty about feeling hostile for not being able to say how I felt, about myself.

F: Sounds to me like you felt trapped?

R: I'd be empty no matter how I responded.

F: How about an even more recent experience – the present—with those feelings?

R: I still feel guilty when I don't feel like filling someone's needs and they expect it. I still feel hostile when I can't express those feelings and have them accepted. I have difficulty often expressing that hostility—I often still fell trapped.

F: Did you see anything new about yourself in that reflection?

R: Yes—I see the trap much clearer. I see where it came from and it feels good to tie that all together. I now have to reevaluate the meaning of the whole experience of having to perform. I have to reevaluate the meaning of hostility for me. I remember that I did express hostility a lot to another aunt that I grew to feel very close to but the aunt that I felt I had to perform for, I never got as close as I wanted. So, it looks like people get closer to each other when they can get closer by expressing hostility and feelings to each other and that the openness of that expression doesn't cause people to go away from each other.

F: Would you like to explore that a little more?

R: Yea—I can see that as a child—not understanding the cause and effect of many things – I defined hostility as the cause of my aloneness. It seems that while the details of my life have changed, my understanding of my self—my feelings—hasn't changed much since I was young. I'm still five years old in some of my feelings about myself.

CARING FOR INSTINCTUAL FEELINGS

The presence of fear, guilt and hostility in our conscious awareness is evidence that our inner somatic feeling center registers empty and that our instinctive needs are not being met. Given this state of our organism, while our guilt may be directed toward ourselves, our fear and the direction of our hostility are projected outward toward any logically convenient source outside of us. Our logic may seem quite bizarre to an observer but to the logic of the empty organism, the projection is a "hook" to hang the blame for our emptiness on a cause outside of us. In moments of emptiness, it is the apparent duty of our thinking to find an obvious source outside and make it responsible until it can find a means to fill our inner self.

Guilt in our awareness derives from several sources that feed it. The somatic feeling of emptiness underlies all of our psychosomatic feelings, or emotional feelings that are a mixture of thinking and feeling. The emotional feeling named *guilt* is interwoven in all our past experiences and is stored, patterned for reuse, in our perceptive process—our intuitions—and colors all present and future experiences with the emptiness that underlies the emotional feeling. Such a coloring of experience presents us with fear in the present and of the future and reduces our spontaneity to life—guilt cuts off our energy in the now. Operating around a basic emptiness, guilt becomes unbearable and we focus it into anger by projecting on others the blame for our condition. This only serves to further reduce our possibilities of using our time meaningfully with others and prevents our needs from being filled—it chases people away and robs us of the possibility of acceptance in our use of time.

The presence of guilt seems to be responsible for our inner awareness of isolation and alienation from other members of the human family. Its presence in us actually drives us further away from our needs satisfaction by spatially separating us from others. Thus both our time and space awareness is empty due to the presence of our guilt.

If we are able to do anything about our emptiness, we must deal with our inner sources of guilt in reflection on past experience before present and future time or space can have any new value to us as an organism relative to those guilt sources. The presence of the inner feeling of emptiness directs our attention to a past experience of guilt and to our inner feeling awareness of the cause in the past. We must be sensitive to that feeling and accept it in order to chase down the cause, ferret it out, reassess the value of the experience to us in order not to further project the blame in anger outward to an external cause. We must look inside of our selves for the cause of our guilt in time past, not outward in space in the present. We carry our feelings about ourselves on into time and events and, in the final analysis; we must take responsibility for them ourselves.

No one else can take responsibility for our feelings—we can neither project that responsibility on others nor can they assume it even though they may seem to want to do so. If we try to make others or if we let others have the responsibility for our feelings, it is only a matter of time until we are forced back on ourselves to deal with and understand them (the feelings). We may try to deny our feelings, as we often do, or avoid those who remind us of them, but in either case we end up further with the feeling of being alone, empty and more confused about our feelings. Like our shadow, our feelings are always with us, cast by us in yet another situation to appear in time.

Our emotional feelings are our self-image. They represent the impact of experience on us and are the historical record of our awareness up through time from birth to the present. Our feelings do not represent our awareness of others but they represent our awareness of ourselves in relation to others—the impact of experience with others.

THE MEANINGFUL USE OF TIME

The closer we feel to another person, the more we want the time we spend together to be full of meaning. *Full of meaning* means that we can open ourselves to another so completely that we can share our instinctual feelings with them spontaneously without giving up the total responsibility of our own feelings. We want to share our instinctual feelings without implying in the sharing that anyone but ourselves needs to take on any responsibility for logical cause or effect connected with the details of that feeling.

The modern human dilemma is that experience has taught us to see possible positions that others might take if we tell them how we feel. And we allow this logic to invade the expression of the feeling, thus distorting the meaning we need to convey. The meaning we need to convey in expressing our instinctive feelings is only to tell others how we feel about ourselves—so we can have the feeling that someone accepts us and cares. What we are afraid of in sharing such natural feelings is that others will try to assume the responsibility for our feelings and make us feel guilty for feeling the way we do. Other things we do with our time seems to be filler—less meaningful activity—to take up the time until we can share ourselves with someone with whom we can be open to the experience of caring.

The whole dilemma is in the present. Its impact is now! But the things we see—sights of the present—resonate with sights of past experiences to color the now. The sounds we hear ring in our ears with sounds of the past and garble the message we hear in the present. The smells in the now remind us of the smells in the past and responses to them. Tastes in the current events are pregnant with those of our past and we salivate to the expectation of past experiences as well. When we touch in the now, we touch to find what is new as well as what has been before. Our whole being responds at this moment to the sum of the meaning of time that has gone before. And the experience of the current event reveals the total impact of the events of the past. We instinctively know all of this and use this awareness naturally. We also know this logically. But to know intellectually is not for us the understanding that frees us to freshly go at life with the vitality we once could experience. And unless we can find and revive the natural zest for life we once could feel, we tend to give up in fear, guilt, and hostility.

To go back and sift through the experiences of our past at first seems a futile search through the trash of days gone by. All of this we have unsuccessfully tried to put behind us. We have often spoken with pride about our ability to live for the now and the future. But the empty feeling in our gut, which we tried to ignore even while we spoke, was a grim private reminder of the unfinished business of the past that was sucking up energy we needed to handle the present.

To go back and explore the instinctual feelings—the impact of experiences—the feelings we felt at the time that was expressed to no one, is not a futile wallowing in the past. Such a reflection on the instinctive feelings, without the emphasis on the details, is to discover for the first time the real meaning of experience. Such reflection builds toward a useful understanding on the now and sets future possibilities in focus for new and exciting life experiences.

The now is the most complicated time of our lives for it contains all of the past, as well as, the new dimensions of the present. If we don't understand the meaning of the past to ourselves, we cannot know the meaning of what is happening now. If the meaning of the past is set in a meaning borrowed from an outside authority, we see no meaning and are empty because of it. If we want the present to be full for us, then we must reassess the past in terms of meaning to ourselves and reject the meaning of any other authority. Not until we can experience this new perspective of the qualities of our instinctive self, are we able to use the present and certainly the future, to fill ourselves as human beings. We may assume such a responsibility and authority for our past, even though we have never consciously assumed such authority in the past. And to take charge in the present requires that we understand that we were in charge in the past, even though we weren't conscious of it when it happened. Our human instinctive qualities, our somatic feelings, were in charge even though we were not conscious of it and we were in charge on an instinctual level when we were born and have been in charge every moment in spite of all the outside evidence to the contrary. A careful exploration through reflection on our gut feelings of *how it felt to be* is a most convincing experience of validation of the above statement.

ANATOMY OF FEELINGS

The idea that instinctive feelings are important to us and that the record of instinctive feelings might be the most accurate record of our lives, requires further understanding of the source of feelings. Such a source must be beyond our early psychological or mental awareness. Instinctive feelings must be available to each of us as newborn babies or even as a prenatal organism. These basic instinctive feelings must be few in number and quite simple to explain.

One concept of the source and nature of basic instinctive feelings that stands the test of reflection in our lives, both in the author's reflections and in reflecting with hundreds of our patients, centers on the basic gut responses felt in each of our earliest recollections. Such gut responses seem to be located in a most interesting way near to the umbilical cord entrance to the organism and close to the point where the major respiratory, digestive, and circulatory components of the life processes exist. Such a response center existing in the unborn or newborn organism that is serviceable to regulate feelings of well being or ill-being prior to psychological awareness seems to be located in the gut region. Given a response center in that region of the gut, we can expect to be aware of signals of fullness and emptiness quite early in life, and such signals produce positive or negative feelings on the state of the organism prior to psychological awareness or thinking awareness. Whether, in fact, such is the case in early prenatal and newborn life is, of course, only conjecture; but we do know, from our own experience with reflection on our feelings and with the vast experience of reflection with our patients, that quite early in our memories our somatic well-being was indicated by a feeling of fullness or emptiness in the pit of the stomach.

We, along with the people with whom we have reflected, have become conscious through our somatic reflections, what the fullness and emptiness gut responses have meant and that certain conditions existed in the context of what was going on around us at the time we first had the feelings. We also have observed, from our own reflections, that these feelings are separated by a sense of time that we knew early in life as internal time relative possibly to the heartbeat close to our gut. The case for when and how a response center of feeling of time is developed is for others to decide, but we do know in our selves—through our feelings—that we can trust to tell ourselves the fullness and emptiness of life that comes from the gut region. We can also say from our own experience of ourselves, that such instinctive somatic responses are not always in concert with our thinking intelligence or head response, but are more reliable in directing our basic human activity than our heads. Such a reliability is especially true when we realize that our psychological response center is trained early for the convenience of others who may not have known or cared about our instinctive feelings.

Feelings that adults know seem to have many names. Feelings that babies know or young children know and respond to are surely less complex and need no naming. With reflection on feelings back in early childhood, years 3, 4, and 5 years old, prior to a time when all the adult names of feelings could have been known, we find an interesting continuity of the record of feeling of emptiness and fullness that helps us remember our authentic selves and tells us how-it-felt-to-be-then. Such feelings tell us how it was to live then in relation to persons, places, things and situations that were important then and often are important to us now because they are still operational and useful to us, as well telling us which ones were not useful then and must be reevaluated in the light of a new day.

The record of our basic instinctive somatic feelings seems to be an accurate record of the fullness and emptiness of our lives. Reflecting upon this feeling record, we find the early variables of our personality that seem to operate in an effort to procure for us more of the fullness feeling and less of the emptiness feeling. While these variables occur in the early record of our feelings, they still exist in the patterns of our present experience. As a young child, we find that we seemed to have operated more directly from the basic instinctive feelings in order to obtain those things that were perceived to satisfy the needs that would bring fullness. When such efforts were frustrated, as young infants and small children, we express openly our feelings by crying. If crying brings no results, we learn to use other subtle means to get what we want or need. As we learn what works, we begin to devise more sophisticated patterns of behavior that give us the feeling of fullness. When we find nothing but emptiness is available to us, we begin to feel of less worth to ourselves. Such emptiness, however, often results in seemingly bizarre attempts to break out and obtain fullness. If over a long period of time, we fail ourselves and are unable to find fullness, we abandon ourselves and borrow a system from some other source to try to make fullness come in some way. Operating on some borrowed outside principle, in order to gain the feeling of fullness or to avoid the feeling of emptiness, we often forget what our basic instinctive somatic feelings are and the result is generally not satisfying or healthy.

We have found in our own reflections that it was not until we came up short in come crisis that we were reminded that we seemed no longer to know who we were or what our purpose for being was. As we reflect back through our lives on our feelings, we can see periods of time when we were busy operating on some external idea of who we were or what our purpose was while our gut was busy registering emptiness. It is in reflection that we can remember the empty feeling and now know how strange our behavior must have seemed to those close to us. There was no way that they could have known what our basic feelings were during those times because our perception was that our feelings were not acceptable and were not spoken. We learned as children that what we felt was not acceptable or we thought that was the case from what we heard or saw around us. It seemed as though we were all playing roles based upon our instinctive somatic feelings but they were distorted by our psychological awareness that probably was not able to identity the emptiness felt in our stomachs. Such was the manner in which we each learned to ignore our basic instinctive feelings and began to let thinking borrowed from others steer the course of our lives. There were many times, we can see now in reflection, that the accurate feeling record was there but the happenings around those feelings were head-trips trying to obtain the fullness that an open expression of the emptiness to someone who cared might have satisfied. Many times, we see now in reflection, that we were lost but somehow never completely. Fortunately, the crisis after crisis that we encounter reminds us that we had lost contact with our selves. These crises were the signs in our lives that our instinctive somatic responses are provided to remind our thinking head that it was taking us away from our selves. This is so in spite of the agony we felt at times when we had to abandon the role that our heads enjoyed playing.

We had a patient, Anne, who came to us in deep distress mid school semester. She was an "a" student and was sure that her chosen field of nursing was exactly what she needed, but she was not able to function in school as she was devastated by a divorce that had just hit her like as she said, "an ocean of waves of sorrow". We had found with our patients that divorce was a time that all of the person's negative feelings of loss from past experiences would crash in on them and while it seemed that all the sadness was related to the loss of the present day spouse, the devastation they were feeling was much bigger and reached far back into their past experiences. While it does not take the sting of divorce away completely, it does help lessen the pain to work on the past unresolved issues and at least erases much of the pain and suffering mixed into one's feelings in the present. Often the person is not even conscious of having the past suffering as it has all been repressed and so well hidden from the conscious ego in our unconscious, our shadow. Once the unconscious content has been brought to light, people would often find that the repression was at least part of the reason the present relationship was not fully functioning and had met with an end. It is often the part of ourselves that we are hiding from our loved one that is the most appealing part of ourselves and holds the key to our feeling pulse that gives energy and life to both ourselves and to our relationship.

As we began in coaching to have her focus on her feelings of sadness, Anne was able to trace it back to the death and loss of her younger brother in childhood. She had been quite young and had, in the way that children often do in absence of information, blamed herself because she had scolded him to get out of her room earlier in the day before his untimely accident attempting to cross the street alone at three years old. Upon reflection on her feelings, she realized that she was not even home at the time the accident occurred and a baby sitter had been in charge of her brother. She felt for the first time in her life a relief that her brother's death was not her fault and was astounded that she was feeling all of that loss and guilt in the present mixed in her feelings of loss of her spouse to an impending divorce. She went home and shared this feeling experience with her spouse and while they finally did part ways, it was as friends and Anne was able to stop blaming herself and continue school successfully to become a nurse. We saw her on several occasions in the halls after the session and noticed that even though she was struggling with a divorce, she possessed a glow and less stress facial expressions about her that had not been there previously.

As we learn to reflect on our feelings, we can see more clearly that each crisis in our lives alerted us to an awareness that we needed to back off the direction we were headed and go back to pick up the signals from our guts and follow them to fullness. As we learn more to do this, we find our thinking less likely to borrow a role from the world for us to play and more likely to work in support of our gut feelings to bring the feeling of fullness to ourselves and live a full and healthy life.

LEVELS OF FEELING

People commonly experience the awareness of feelings as a combination of logic and feeling rather than a purely instinctive gut feeling of necessity. The inner instinctive feeling is surely there but our conscious awareness is so distracted toward the outside situation through our senses that the instinctive human feelings are available to us only in a combined form with some outside authoritative thinking we have accepted. This type of common feeling experience or level of feeling consciousness may be called psychosomatic feelings in contrast to the purely instinctive somatic feelings of the human organism.

We experience the psychosomatic level of feeling to be allied with our attachments to outside authority. In situations where we are conscious of the importance of what other's think or how we perform, we become aware that our basic feelings are set side-by-side with the logic of the external authority in the situation and we tend to judge our position in terms of that outside view. Invariably, we come up short and lose in that comparison. We experience the tendency of the logic to judge this type of feeling position to be weak and unreliable. The weakness seems to be related to the logical compromise of our instinctive feelings. Compromised feelings are inevitably unreliable because in such a situation we find we are strung-out away from ourselves. From the point of view of the Self, we find in reflecting on what is important to us that it was the logic system that we accepted that were unreliable. We find it always unreliable to accept outside principles that do not satisfy the instinctual feelings when we apply them to our inner needs.

It is helpful to remember that if the feeling is named—fear, hostility, guilt, jealousy, joy, sadness, etc.—it is not a basic instinctive feeling since the act of naming by the logic system attaches the feeling to an outside judgment even though it is related to emptiness or fullness on the inside of us. And it is the inner instinctive feelings with which we need to deal not the outside person, situation or thing with which the named feeling is associated. Often the outside situation is not even a real factor with which we can deal. We can project on a host of fantasies in the outside world while the real problem lies deep in our inner instinctive feelings of necessity.

BECOMING AWARE OF INSTINCTIVE FEELINGS

As you reflect on your instinctive feelings, you may remember feeling at times empty and alone—wondering if everyone felt that way. And not having feedback from others you may even have surmised that most other people must not feel the way you do. The following is a revised excerpt from our original book, *Born of the Human Family*,[2] in which we included a personal account of how we became aware of our own instinctive feelings. We originally wrote much of the book in the first person, "I", to demonstrate how the authors discovered instinctive gut feelings and to assist the reader in identifying with the material in their own feeling awareness.

> *I can personally even remember watching other people, trying to decide who felt empty and who felt full. It seemed that certain situations caused some to feel empty, and other people not*

to feel empty. In other situations the reverse seemed not to be true for the same people. I thought that there must be some way I would not have to feel empty since there were always some who seemed to feel all right about them Selves.

I could not tell by looking at the outside of people if any were feeling the way I felt. I conjectured that most people felt in control. I wanted to feel that way too. I did not want to feel emptiness. So I tried all kinds of things not to feel the emptiness. This started way back when I was a young child. These things I did were things my head told me to do, to get away from the emptiness. I even copied some things others were doing that looked like they would be fulfilling. With my head—my upper brain—I tried to reason the emptiness in terms that I also picked up from other people. My head defined my emptiness, in certain situations, as patterns—hostility, guilt, and fear. Always it was my rational description of my emptiness—the source of reason for the feeling was defined as one outside of my Self.

It seems like our logic was saying that my emptiness was there because the world was not living up to my expectations or that I was not living up to the world's expectations of me. In other words, I was coming up short—less than— because of something or someone outside of my Self.

When my head said my emptiness was because of my Self, it named the feeling guilt. My head named my emptiness hostility or fear if it attributed the source to a situation or person outside. And these judgments came from other people outside of my Self. I can remember trying all kinds of things my head said would get rid of the emptiness because emptiness was not a feeling I should have. Emptiness was not comfortable or necessary to feel as a human being. I tried all kinds of things to get rid of the feelings—but I never could. I could experience a temporary feeling of happiness, when I did something successfully that my head said would get rid of the emptiness, but happiness was only temporary. The emptiness was still there and I had to use more and more energy to get away from the awareness of the emptiness inside of me. After making many unsuccessful attempts at getting away from the awareness of my emptiness, I began to feel a hopelessness of achieving any real fullness by letting my head lead the way out of emptiness. If I could not accept my empty feeling, it seemed hopeless.

At certain times in my life other people would come to me and say they understood my feelings. I would show my empty feelings a little and withdraw in from others until I shared my empty feelings with a few other people who accepted my feelings completely. Then there was not the same need to get away from my empty feelings. At that point, I could begin to be a little quieter with my Self and begin to feel through life. I began to feel more aware of my feelings of empty or full as they happened. I felt less of a need to put my empty feelings down or get away from the awareness of them. To deny them was no longer necessary. It gradually became possible to look at the judgments my head had made and re-evaluate its meanings and see if in my gut my emptiness was really caused by what my head said was the cause. I began wanting to take more responsibility for my feelings. And I was more willing to take more responsibility for my feelings. I was more willing to experience my feelings and to accept my own Self as the source rather than project it on the outside world. I began not putting my Self down. I realized that what is inside me is good— all of it! So, accepting my gut feelings—my Self— began with a process of letting my head take over—using judgments of the world around me— and finding emptiness in all directions, until I had to turn around and go back to the source of my very being—my instinctive feelings [of emptiness and fullness in the gut]. Until I could accept my emptiness enough to express it and have my feelings accepted by another as perfectly human— I felt imperfectly human. When a car is out of gas, we do not assign a negative value to the car for being empty. But when a human being is empty, the cultural idea seems to be to assign a negative value to the person. Being empty is simply a signal to me. It is not really good or bad—it is in every human and tells us something very important about our Selves.

One night, after I realized that all my empty feeling was a signal to be felt and heard and not denied—not to get strung-out in my head away from—I had an interesting experience with fear. I was feeling fear. I remember thinking—well, I can either rationalize it away, try to do something that my head says will help prevent the fear or let my Self feel it and get into it. I said to my Self that it is okay to feel fear. In fact, it might be a signal telling me something other than what my head says it is. Maybe the fear is not really telling me that something outside of me is going to hurt me. Maybe my fear comes from an inner source, which I could understand. Maybe I could understand my Self through this feeling my head calls fear. And then I could clearly understand it. As a matter of fact, the feeling of fear was closer to emptiness once my head was turned off.

When my head is going and I fear—I feel intensity in my head that goes out to infinity— infinite possibilities of fear that I cannot deal with. But as I drop my analysis of the fear and concentrate on the feeling of the fear, it is so close to emptiness that it feels like all other feelings of emptiness. It is at that point that I can see what I am really empty about. I am really not afraid— there is nothing real to be afraid of—I am just empty. Fear is just something that my head has said is a reason for my emptiness. A lot of times my emptiness is related to something very much in my present experience of the day or the day before. Usually, my emptiness relates to the sharing or lack of sharing of instinctive feeling with people that I live closely with. My head goes wild with my emptiness and really gets me strung out [in thoughts that are ungrounded in the reality around me]. What my head does is produce anxiety. It projects so many possibilities that it makes dealing with fear impossible.

The one thing that overcomes that emptiness is reaching out to someone with my emptiness— expressing the emptiness. Reflecting back over the past with feelings to understand and share my emptiness with another person helps to support the Self and lessens the need for head-trips in the present. The feeling-reflection process helps me

> *stay simple in understanding my Self—*
> *understanding my emptiness and fullness—and*
> *my need to share myself with others.*
>
> *It seems that I show my empty feelings to*
> *people a little at a time. I seem to pop out and*
> *back in—coming out a little further each time. I*
> *know that I do not fully accept my empty feelings*
> *until another person shows me that they have the*
> *same feelings and we share our emptiness*
> *together. Then I feel really full [in this*
> *communication with another member of the*
> *human family].*

We have found with our many patients and ourselves that once we become aware of the fullness of sharing, there is a great drive to sustain it. Even though we can tolerate the emptiness and realize it is an important human signal that directs us toward our purpose for being, we want to be full. Accepting the emptiness as an important signal does not mean that we wallow in the empty feeling alone. As a matter of fact, there is a tremendous drive to reach out to others and share instinctive feelings once we accept our own as important signals.

STRUCTURED AWARENESS OF FEELINGS

The psychosomatic feelings, such as hostility, fear, guilt, sadness, and joy, are an attempt by our logic to name the source of the instinctive somatic feeling of emptiness or fullness in the gut. While there are an infinite number of psychosomatic feelings as there are an infinite number of possible logical projections, they are all based on the instinctive somatic feelings of emptiness and fullness.

There is a need to understand our psychosomatic feelings in terms of instinctive somatic inner feelings rather than terms of outer logical authority. Outer authority is so vague and diverse as to cover—complicate our understanding—and it draws attention away from our selves and focuses attention on those things that are only perceived through outer sense experience—sight, sound, taste, touch, and smell. The sensing capacity is so strong that the inner feeling signals are easy to ignore until we reach a crisis point. Understanding the structure of psychosomatic feelings in terms of inner instinctive feelings is designed to build the bridge between our inner and outer worlds to avoid a crisis.

When our psychosomatic feelings are understood in relation to our instinctive somatic feelings, then we can begin to take the responsibility for our Selves to each fulfill our inherent-purpose-for-being. The sections on the following pages identify the basic psychosomatic feelings as signals leading to an awareness of the process of discovery of our inner-Self signals.

Hostility

Hostility erupts when we have accepted an external judgment, which is in conflict with our instinctive human feelings, and we have established an intuitive role—an operating base away from our feeling center—in order to deal with the external judgment until a resolution is made of the conflict or to avoid making a resolution of the internal conflict.

Some of the blame for the way we feel is often projected on the outside authority. A few such typical projections will probably be familiar. I feel hostile towards:

"those who make me feel guilty"

" those who make me feel small"

"those who don't care about me"

'those who take advantage of me"

"those who make me feel negative about myself in
any way"

"those who remind me I'm a phony"

"those things that make me feel stupid"

Hostility seems to be defense energy provided for an indefensible role in the world we have assumed to protect ourselves against exposing our instinctive feeling of emptiness; never is it associated with the instinctive feeling of fullness.

When we are operating in an assumed role, we take on that role because our inner Self is empty relative to the situation in which we assume the role and we strive always for fullness. The role or roles we assume are intuitive models based on that which we have perceived of the outer world—the roles for which we perceive the need (mostly through sight and sound). The role we assume may be a conscious role as wife, husband, student, teacher mother, father or a less conscious role as lover, friend, savior, saved one, sinner, slave or many other suitable ideas of what a person might be or should be. When we commission our logic to assume a role based upon an outside judgment or principle, our gain is not likely or necessarily related to the fullness of our Self. Our logic has done its job—to tell us what others think we should do—but the reality of the results may not coincide with the expectation for fullness provided by our intuition because our intuition does not take our present Self into consideration. If inner fullness does not result from an event according to the role prescription, our logic is faced with failure and is likely to project the cause on the one from whom we have accepted the judgment and towards whom we maintain the role. In all of this surface management, our inner Self remains empty.

It is almost as though our inner Self assumes that our logic is working for it and furnishes energy to the logic for the purpose of providing for its needs. If our logic has been distracted by outside pressure and fails to provide for our inner Self, the energy furnished for fulfillment of our inner Self is squandered by the logic in the form of hostility in defense of its assumed role position. If the logic is, in fact, working directly for our inner instinctive feelings, the energy for the situation is used for fulfillment and no hostility is experienced. Most of us, who have found our Selves playing a role over a period of time, know how exhausting it is to maintain it.

The roles assumed by our logic in childhood, with which we may still operate as an adult, may be buried deep in lower levels of our awareness. It appears as though our logic can forget the material it has operated with—external principles used and accepted early in our lives. It seems that our logic has no memory of the roles it has played. But the experience gained from using the early roles in our lives are still available from our intuition in the form of expectations, and is processed by our logic whenever the adult situation calls for it. If the early role models were in conflict with our instinctive feelings at the time they were used, they still seem to produce the same conflicts—whether or not we are aware of it. We have found that behind all anger, there is guilt and the guilt relates to not being able to defend oneself in an indefensible role we have assumed out of emptiness.

Very often we become aware that we feel negative about our Self but we do not know why. Certain situations seem to produce such feelings more than others. Thinking about the cause produces no logical reason. But reflecting on the feeling—chasing it back to earlier times when we remember feeling the same before—we can become aware of a role assumed in childhood when our feelings of emptiness about an issue were not accepted. It is necessary to have the experience of sharing together and exchanging these empty feelings with another person, in order to totally accept our Self and become totally responsible for our Self.

Guilt

As a child, we often felt empty and alone. To try to overcome these feelings, we reach out to explore in the outside world, trying to find someone who would understand and accept the way we feel inside our Self. We may invent bizarre things to do to attract people to us. But often the effect is the opposite of what we expected and we are scolded for not caring [mother or father]. As we accept the judgment for not caring about others, we may feel the pangs of guilt—and later as we identify this feeling our head picks up from our culture the name of the feeling we receive as *guilt*.

The following is a revised excerpt from our earlier book *Born of the Human family*[3], in which the authors describe the discovery of the process of experiencing guilt as a child and into adulthood, and how the judgments from others accepted in this guilt led to further emptiness, stress, and inner conflict:

> *My real inner instinctive feelings of emptiness and aloneness I could not share with anyone—I could not seem to tell anyone how empty and alone I felt. There seemed to be a role I had not yet learned that would make me acceptable to others in the outside world and take away my emptiness.*
>
> *As I assumed role after role from external expectations and pressures, there developed an internal conflict between my thinking and my instinctive feelings. I would accept what others*

told me I should do, meanwhile my inner feelings were ignored, and inevitably, I would end up empty and alone again.

I would seem to come up short—my Self never seemed to be acceptable as I was. I was expected to perform one way in a role but another way seemed more acceptable if I cared about my feelings. Such an assumed external judgment against my own instinctive feelings made me feel empty. What others wanted of me in a role and wanted me to accept was not really me. If I did not perform because of my instinctive feelings, the outside judgment was present in my awareness before I refused or maybe it would come in on me in the actual experience. And the tendency was for my logic to say that my emptiness was because I felt less than in the role—I had not lived up to the model of a good person and I felt guilty. The relationship of the guilt to my emptiness was that I had accepted an outside judgment and came up short.

Alone. The reason I came up short feeling negative alone—less than my judgment said I should—I was still empty. The reason I came up short feeling negative about my Self was that I could not share my feelings of emptiness with anyone in relation to the initial expectations of the role.

However, I could not go against my instinctive feelings for long without coming up short eventually. Even though I may be a big success in the eyes of the observing world in the role I have accepted, I experience no fullness inside if I deny my instinctive feelings in accepting the role. At the point where I come up short in the role, I have realized that I have not followed my instinctive feelings and yet I am willing to give up the role and be my true Self. I feel guilty if I try to follow my instinctive feelings, but at the same time, accept the external judgment that I should have performed differently. My problem is that I want to be my Self and, at the same time, I want to be accepted by the outside world. If my experience is that my instinctive feelings are unacceptable by the world and yet I must follow my feelings to be me, I feel guilty because I am less than that which is acceptable—empty and alone. In this state of inner conflict, I usually do poorly in a role and feel more empty and alone from the negative judgments I am getting.

Our inner needs seem to be to accept our instinctive feelings as valid for a human being and to seek to share the emptiness we feel in relation to the outside world with someone who cares. Guilt is an inaccurate statement of the inner instinctive feelings. It is a compromise of the instinctive feelings caused by acceptance of an external judgment by our logic presumably to aid us in reaching our pay-off. Such a compromise rarely works for long and seldom, if ever, results in any permanent gratification. Immediate satisfaction or happiness may result, but no true Self-acceptance or growth toward inner fullness takes place. It is not until we are able to share our inner feelings—exchange the instinctive feelings of where we are as a person—with another person, that we can accept our true Self, reject external judgments and roles, perform according to our inner instinctive feelings and not feel guilty.

Fear

Fear is a psychosomatic response reflecting our inner instinctive feelings against a perceived danger. When we are afraid, our logic is focused on our sense experience, telling us that there is a condition out there with which we are inadequate to deal. The psychosomatic feeling being experienced is related to the instinctive feeling of emptiness within us. Our logic generally tries to project the fear onto the situation rather than take the responsibility for the feeling of emptiness and we judge our selves inadequate to cope.

If we are in a boat in a storm and afraid, the fear does not come from the situation but from the underlying emptiness in our aloneness that we have not shared with another person. There may be some real danger in coping with the situation but the fear, which we experience, is not produced by that danger. The danger is the trigger of our inner feelings. The feeling of fear that wells up in us always relates to an inner feeling of emptiness previously experienced. The "gut knot" accompanying the fear is the somatic response to the emptiness, not the fear of the immediate danger.

The fear indicates that we have had some specific experiences in our lives in which we have felt empty but the feeling was not accepted or perceived to be shared by others. Instead of being able to share the empty feeling with someone who would accept it, we have accepted the judgment that we are less than for feeling empty and inadequate to deal alone. These judgments, accumulated over a period of time, are triggered by a current event in our life and cave-in on us.

Very often we find that because we have judged our Self less than and incapable for feeling empty, we have given the responsibility for ourselves to some person, situation or principle (perhaps religious ideals) outside of our Self and in that specific way we have lost control. When the authority person or situation is absent or perceived as powerless as we are to cope, we are afraid and we are reminded that we have emptied our Self. It is as though we have been hiding behind a more adequate protector of our Self than we are naturally. When the protection is taken away, we are left alone and empty. Rather than indicating an outside danger over which we have no control, fear is a necessary signal that indicates there is some emptiness inside of us that has not been shared and exchanged with another person.

The following is a recent account of how the feeling of fear as a flag of an underlying feeling of emptiness was discovered by one of the authors.

> *I began to realize that fear had little to do with the outside situation or object that I feared and more to do with my own emptiness when I lived in Florida and we would have hurricanes. Some days there would be an announcement that a hurricane was possibly on the way to our town and I would be in a complete panic. I felt like I was going to be completely overcome, my whole family wiped out and death was impending. But in truth, it may not have been much of a possibility that it was even coming our way at all and it may have been a very small hurricane. Then another week, an announcement would come of an approaching hurricane, a much bigger one than the last and much more likely to hit our town. But surprisingly, I would barely care about it and go about my day, taking some hurricane safety precautions, but otherwise acting and feeling as if it was nothing to worry about.*
>
> *I found this difference in reaction very curious and after experiencing this random fear versus*

calmness in the face of danger; I began to reflect on my feelings on those days. As I felt through the days I had these experiences, I could see that on the days I feared the hurricanes, feared my death and the death of others, there was always an underlying emptiness, with which I came into the experience. And the emptiness had to do with how close I felt to others and how in control of my own responses I was already feeling in my normal life just prior to the hurricane announcement. The hurricane was then just a trigger event and my fear was a signal that I was already feeling empty and out of control on a deeper level of feeling. Sharing this with another human being who could accept my feelings generally relieved the fear and I could focus successfully without panic on taking proper precautions needed for hurricane safety and felt a relief of stress.

Joy

The psychosomatic feeling of joy is experienced when our expectations are met or more than met in a situation. Expectations are set up around roles provided by the external world. The feeling of joy is the experience of role fulfillment rather than the acceptance of the condition of my inner self—the feeling of emptiness or fullness alone.

If we are striving to fill an expectation of a role, for instance, as being a good wife, and we meet the expectation by cooking a good dinner, then our head says "I am okay because I satisfied the world's judgment of me" and we feel a temporary joy. We often see in reflection of the experience that the basic model of expectation was not directed toward our inner needs as a person and has not altered our real inner feelings in any way toward fullness.

The following is an excerpt from our earlier book *Born of the Human Family*,[4] in which the author speaking describes the inner discovery of how following the joy of fulfilling a role can lead to a crisis in one's life.

> *When I was very young, I felt empty and alone. The expectation from the outer world was that, if I would just learn to spell and read then I would be acceptable and feel differently. I pushed my Self to learn to perform [in school] for years. And then finally, when I experienced meeting my expectation of a good student, I experienced a temporary joy. But I was still alone and empty inside, as the empty feeling had not been accepted by my Self or the outer world. I was trying to be accepted for what others thought I should do, not for what I experienced my Self to be. It was not until my instinctive feelings were in conflict with the role, that I questioned performing the role of good student. At the point of awareness of my internal conflict, the temporary joy became a negative feeling and was burdensome because of my instinctive feelings. The feeling of joy encouraged me to accept the role but my inner feelings denied the value of it. The pressure of the joy, which encouraged me to be more successful and take on more and more expectations, was in conflict with my instinctive feelings. The instinctive feelings did not support the external role with the energy demanded and eventually I become exhausted and aware of my emptiness. It is crucial at this point that I accept my emptiness as an important signal of my inner needs and reject the negative external judgment of my Self*

for not fulfilling the roles. If I accept the external judgment on my Self, I may come up fighting again to fulfill another external expectation, but in so doing I am vulnerable to experience a greater crisis later on. It is through my experience of crisis after crisis in my life that I have seen the relationship between my instinctive inner feelings to the temporary psychosomatic feeling of joy.

We once had a patient who was a renowned stain glass artist in his locality. While extremely successful both artistically and economically, he expressed that he was so very empty from his work. And upon reflection on his feelings, he found that he had begun his career early in life and was so rewarded positively by his family that he kept doing it, even though he was not fulfilled on an instinctive gut feeling level by his work. Marrying and having children only added to his pressure to succeed in a career and it seemed to make it all the more impossible for him to stop a successful career as a stain glass artist. At the time we saw him, he was and had been working for years in a career that emptied him and he had never found the opportunity to stop his work and make a career change, although he now desperately wanted to do so. He was beginning to experience medical symptoms that he intuitively felt related to working in a career that he wanted to walk away from. Yet he was frightened to make a career change and somewhat frozen in his effort to do so. Upon reflection on his feelings, we were able to trace his fear of leaving the career back to early childhood demands upon his performance from his well-meaning parents. After several sessions, he was able to understand the source of his fear of change, gain the awareness of his true instinctual needs, and then make a career change into a business field he choose that was more truly satisfying for him. And he was able to use his knowledge of the field of art in his new business of buying and selling art and this continuity was quite fulfilling for him. And by the way, the last time we heard from him after his career change, we understand that he does voluntarily still make stain glass, but on a limited bases that fits his own inner need time-schedule of production rather than outer demands for performance success.

WHEN CARING EXISTS

Many of you would agree that caring in an intimate relationship presents the greatest challenge to you in maintaining control of your own responses to life and feeling acceptance for it. The closer we get to another member of the human family, in both time and space, the more familiar we must become with our inner needs and with theirs. Such familiarity requires a spontaneity and openness with feelings for which we have had little support and experience. If we are going to show another person the caring that supports life and health in a relationship, we must learn quickly a new way of viewing our Self and the other person that is different from our training as children and even as adults up until this moment.

The art of caring presents our minds with a confusing paradox. If we can spend our time taking care of our instinctive needs and trust those needs, if we can let others spend their time taking care of their instinctive needs and trust those needs, then we are laying the foundation for an intimate relationship that will grow and survive. The fear is that we will grow apart, but the contrary is true, since we can only feel truly loved for who we truly are and that requires that we do not hide our feelings under behavior that we force upon ourselves to conform to our understanding of who we should be to sustain a relationship.

If we logically pursue a relationship according to some acceptable set of rules, and in the process ignore our inner needs, either of us, we will end up feeling empty and with no serviceable relationship for either of us. We will have set a direct course towards a crisis in our lives. Often, a crisis of health issues is our body' s way of surfacing these pressing needs and comes after a long relationship of giving up the caring of our own feelings in favor of assuming a role or multiple roles and behaving in what we see as responsible ways for a wife, husband, son, daughter, mother, father, in-law, etc. The paradox seems to be that attention to the details of the relationship tends to make it more important than the persons in it. Paying attention to the persons and their inner needs, bonds the relationship that serves the needs of both persons. By paying attention to the important ingredients— the feelings and the stuff a relationship is made of, rather than the form—an intimate caring relationship is created.

Centering on the inner needs of personhood is not an easy task and it flies in the face of traditions, both Eastern and Western. The work involved often feels constantly uphill, often agonizing and frightening. The only incentive for taking such a bold course of action is that we are weary of letting crises dictate our use of time—often having to dig our way out of one crisis after another. By taking the responsibility for our feelings and directing our attention to what is important to our feeling center, we determine the use of time and minimize the fateful crisis. Instead of coming out of the past with guilt, looking into the future with fear, while loosing the value of the now and feeling angry about it, we can begin to understand the responsibility we have always had to our instinctive nature. We need not feel guilty for the necessity of acceptance and we need not feel guilty for taking control of our time to find acceptance.

If there is any validity to the concept of instinctive necessity and that somatic feelings of empty-full in the gut indicate the state of the organism in relation to basic needs satisfaction, then caring about our Selves and caring about another person derives its meaning from the inner awareness of the nature of the organism. And if there is any validity to the idea that the sense of guilt awareness precedes our awareness of our Self as individuals—after birth—and that the experience of guilt found in reflection is a compounding of prenatal or postnatal experience, then it is necessary in the relationship between two persons who intend to spend meaningful time together to open such feelings to the other. It is important to take the responsibility for feelings without projection of cause on the other and to make our awareness of guilt available in order for others to take such feelings into account in the relationship. And if there is any validity to the idea that while we all have identical needs within the human family but that we have a schedule of needs satisfaction all our own, then it is not surprising that what seems to be our uniqueness as individuals and even cultures is the style and timing we have developed in early childhood and later in relation to the environment in which we yearn to thrive and satisfy those needs we have when it is necessary for us to do so.

By an awareness of the inner nature and the outer coping style, caring for another becomes looking past the behavior of the other with acceptance for the instinctive needs trying to be met, for this is the only place in our consciousness that we can truly meet another person. This awareness of inner human feeling needs may be particularly valuable in relationships of people from different cultures whose coping styles are vastly different. Our ability to do this depends heavily upon the fullness of our own feelings. If we are empty, we loose our capacity to cope with other's needs and we need to learn to accept this state for our Self and others. When we can be aware of our emptiness and share this feelings spontaneously, we are caring for our selves and beginning to fill our selves from this not-so-simple admission.

The negative self-concept and resulting guilt we carry from early childhood closes down our spontaneity and interferes with the caring experience in the present. Guilt forces us to deal logically on the surface with some learned role to do what appears to be caring. Such caring becomes special, physical, and material, which further compounds the guilt by offering no acceptance or understanding of our inner nature and needs.

To gain the acceptance of our inner instinctive needs, we must deliberately take control of our time and work constantly through the process of reflecting on our inner instinctive somatic feelings so that we can care for and feel cared for by another human being. It is the choice we all face to pursue this inner direction in our living with the constant effort involved rather than to leave caring to the fate of pretending—to the ultimate crisis that role playing will certainly bring.

We offer the charts on the following pages as a summary of what it means to experience caring for our selves and others by working to become closer to the consciousness of our instinctive somatic gut feelings:

WHEN WE CARE:
We care about our Selves, how we feel about ourSelves—and we want to share our feelings about ourSelves .
Instead of projecting judgments on others as the cause of our feelings, we try to look for the source of our feelings inside ourSelves—from our own experience with ourSelves.
We look upon our behavior—the things we have done and do—as an inner necessity at the moment of doing. As we become aware of inner necessity, we learn to accept our every action and the meaning of our actions in terms of our instinctive needs.
We find the beauty and reliability in our instinctive human responses and look for the same beauty in others.
We try to find our Selves—basic human needs—in others.
We feel compassion and understanding of inner needs for ourSelves and for others, and we are free to modify our behavior according to a clearer understanding of the inner needs of ourSelves and others.

WHEN WE FEEL CARING FROM OTHERS:
We feel the possibility of caring from another when we perceive them caring for their own inner needs and feelings.
We feel caring from another when they offer to share their inner feelings with us.
We feel caring from another when they are looking for those same inner feelings in us that they are aware of in themSelves.
We feel caring from another—the most meaningful time for us—when we share our inner feelings and we find the same inner qualities in each other.
We feel caring from another, even in the face of the other's judgments about us, when the other has shared their inner feelings with us and we are aware of how they feel about them Selves.
We feel caring from the other person when they express that they understand their inner needs, and they feel free to modify their behavior according to their new understanding of the needs of themSelves and others

Not for a moment dare we succumb to the illusion that an archetype can be finally explained and disposed of....The most we can do is to dream the myth onwards and give it a modern dress.
(Carl Jung, 1992)

CHAPTER FOUR:

A NEW IMAGE OF HUMAN NATURE

The most passionate occupation of our individual lives has been to test out, tear apart, and then reinvent the myth we learned in early childhood that following our inner nature is unreliable as a guide in making life decisions. We are finding a new way to view others and ourselves as having a strong inner nature that is a reliable center of reference for life decisions and whose strength is never diminished. While it may be necessary for our inner nature to relinquish control overtly, it is covertly guiding us and responding to the state of our organism and the fulfillment of its natural purpose. Our inner nature is always calling to us to be uncovered and followed; and we think that is so for all members of the human family. When we do follow our inner nature, we find that we are more caring for both others, and ourselves and we have more energy available for creative productivity.

ON THE THRESHOLD OF A RENAISSANCE

Myths are organic, alive and teeming with energy of the psyche. We can't expect the old myths to necessarily reveal our plight nor even our Nature. As humanity grows, evolves and changes, new myths are born and in time are buried safely in the veils of our deepest feelings, our instinctive needs carried in our collective unconscious. With the coming of the new paradigm and the new age that humanity is presently moving rapidly toward, our gut brain awareness is emerging as part of a new mythology.

Science has largely been the catalyst of the present evolution of the psyche of humanity. Our need for self-reflection and self-awareness in the last decades was first called to action by our view of the first image of our earth from space. We saw our home for the first time from an external perspective and it was much like looking in a collective mirror for the first time. To see this encompassing image compelled us to reflect on who we are as a whole. No longer could we see ourselves, our humanity, living on our Earth home as separate people living on separate continents, separate countries with separate tribes, separate families, and separate individual people without also realizing that we are also united as Earthlings. We understood viewing this image intuitively if not logically that there is a perspective that is not centered on this planet, but beyond us and larger than us, encompassing us. We could not, up until this time, truly understand in our thinking this larger perspective of which we are that the image of our earth from space brought us. It was not until the astronauts who board the Apollo 8 gave us the image of the first view of earth from space that our understanding of our living planet and ourselves felt truly like an inclusive entity—part of a larger being. Until that time, only a theory brought us the feeling. Now, with the image awareness as well, we can begin to reflect and intuit on a larger scale. With this new global understanding, our humanity might be able to better relate with all of nature on our planet, viewing ourselves as one global entity, and to contemplate what function our humanity might be able to provide for the larger being of the solar system. But to understand what our function might be, we must first reflect on who we really are. And thus, both our new image of ourselves as one global being and the greater awareness of our relationship to the solar system, compels us to begin an Age of Reflection and Discovery about how we operate with our own human nature.

The person with an earth-centered perspective sees oneself as being at the center of his and her universe, creating and disposing of all things at its will. However, the prototype of an evolving people with a new universal perspective, have a different relationship with life. We are becoming star centered and know that we are but a small aspect of a much larger whole. We are beginning to perceive ourselves less as being the central force in the universe with command over other creatures. We are becoming cooperative agents in the ongoing unfolding of a natural plan toward total realization and self-fulfillment of the true nature for all beings. And we as individuals are beginning to not only act for ourselves alone but for all humanity, which means ultimately for the benefit of all sentient beings. Power among evolving humanity comes from accepting responsibility for our own human nature and wisdom comes from encouraging others to do the same. The triumph of the emerging humanity is that we are learning to care more for our loved ones than we do for things and to find joy in helping everyone to succeed. The closer we get to the awareness of our feelings, the nearer we get to self-realization, and the happier we all become. We are learning that we do not need some outer authority to tell us what to do nor do we need them to approve of our endeavors (although few of us proceed very far without the nurturing feedback of others); and that if we act from an inner authority that comes from being in touch with our inner nature, we are caring and benevolently evolving.

Being aware of our instinctive feelings, individually and collectively, is at the very center of the evolving humanity. As we become progressively more and more of our true selves, shedding the layers of dogma, enculturation and just plain confusion and uncertainty, we begin to participate in the formation of a more human culture. We can look to the past to find the roots of our humanity and revive a life once lived or we can craft a new image of humanity now in our own lives and look to the future in which the world is living a life of caring for ourselves and others.

We live on the threshold of a Renaissance in human consciousness. To understand this is soothing and it is necessary to be there in that awareness as soon as possible if we are to thrive during this time. It is a difficult time for people because so many old forms, old thoughts, are breaking up and dissolving in front of our eyes. It is frightening because the old orders are changing and what we once knew about our world and ourselves is changing rapidly.

The idea that we have two brains, not just one in the head but also one in the gut, is unthinkable for many people at first. In 1998, Dr. Michael Gershon, Chairman of the Dept of Pathology and Cell Biology at Columbia University, made a medical breakthrough that demonstrated that we have two distinct brains, one in the Central Nerves System and one in the Enteric Nervous System, the upper brain and the gut brain, respectively. But as we begin to examine what this really means, we see that it gives us a greater ability and potential if used in unison. The old saying that two heads are better than one can be rewritten to say that two brains are better than one and once understood it gives us greater calm and a resolve to create and fulfill our time on earth with meaning and caring for all life. And as we are in contact with our instinctive feelings, bringing the rational head brain of the CNS in service of the needs of the gut brain of the ENS, time is understood as an illusion and there is only the eternally living now, full of life and meaning in the present.

BASIC HUMAN NEEDS

It does not take a college education to realize that our present financial situation exposes the marginalization of the US population—its humanity—in favor of its industrial and financial complex. This is a kind of a trickle-down, water boarding of our instinctual human nature. The country's humanity is starving—dying—while entertainers hold their industries' leashes on our minds so we don't realize that our bodies are being destroyed. We have become so fixated on the environmental trash, that we have lost contact with ourselves. The external environments are establishing the image of our human-ness we accept, rather than by the internal design we have been given by our DNA/RNA.

This intentional daily menu of imitation human need is emptying our lives, making us mentally and physically sick with stress, to the point that we have become dependent upon medical practice and pill peddlers to keep us alive. It shouldn't surprise anyone, who reflects on his own well being, that the demand for health care is driven by the lack of care we take of our selves—our lack of conscious concern for our own individual minds and bodies.

A Renaissance is occurring in the field of neurological medicine, which is beginning to determine what our environments need to be to maintain a healthy mind and body. We are not paying enough attention to the results of that research, which effects us individually, to make the necessary drastic changes. And those necessary changes are getting more challenging every generation. The main reason for this neglect of our selves is that we are faced with having to change the age-old environments that have defined the images of ourselves as humans. And, these images have been taken for granted as the very essence of our being, in spite of much evidence to the contrary. The evidence we are referring to comes from the inner small voice, deep inside the body that is telling us all, that "something isn't right!"

Those who find strength in exploration and experimentation, and are curious to try new ideas for greater comfort in control of their own time and space, welcome change to take control of their destiny—"life may be harsh and we can make it much better." Those who find comfort in the commitments of the past and live in fear that cultural change will upset their promise of a better life in the future, and will resist any basic changes, for, "life may be harsh but it could be much worse." Neither of the two points of view is necessarily accurate unless cultural change has the basic needs of human nature—human instincts—in mind as the objective.

So, what are the basic human needs we are talking about? We each need the Freedom and sense of feeling in control to learn how to express our unique Self, so we can gain attention of genuine Acceptance from our fellow human beings, to thereby, accept one Self—scars and all. We learn this art of consciousness and expression of our basic human needs from the moment we are born until we pass puberty. At this point after puberty, our humanity is complete, and we are prepared to become a member of society as an ethical, yet a unique, loving, caring, sharing, human being.

At the beginning we said, "It doesn't take a college education to realize that our present financial situation exposes the marginalization of the US population—its humanity." That seems to be true! However, without the experience of an education that gets us in touch with our human nature, there won't be enough of us in the college environments who will know how to fix what is wrong.

Therefore, we could go on as we have in the past toward further marginalization of our human-ness.

We mentioned a "small voice" before. The nature of the voice is not necessarily so small, especially when there is a disturbance like a bellyache, constipation or a build-up of gas. The inner voice also speaks quite clearly of its satisfaction with a good meal filling the stomach, or a drink of cool water after a work out. Perhaps it seems small because it does not speak a language like the upper brain, and it is quiet, compared to the brain we know, as it is automatically doing an assigned task of digesting the food we have selected to put in the mouth providing the energy for the entire organic system. Perhaps it seems small compared to the voices from the outside world, voices which ride in through the senses to inform us of the goings-on in the environments outside. On the other hand, we might also say that we experience the voice as an inner feeling, which the upper brain seems to sense only when the body is completely empty and in a condition of stress or completely full and in a condition of wellbeing. Whatever the feeling has seemed to be in the past, it has been a great mystery of the ages to which we offer an exploration and answers to through the awareness and understanding of the intelligence of the gut instincts, along with what this means as a new myth for humanity to follow as a guide in the enlightenment of the 21st century inclusive worldview that is still slowly emerging.

NEEDED: A NEW MYTH FOR HUMANITY THAT REDUCES STRESS

The late great American mythologist and lecturer Joseph Campbell[1] challenged us to explore and create a new myth for humanity. We see that by acknowledging the Enteric

Nervous System in the gut to provide a new image of human nature, a new myth of humanity also emerges.

The old myth of who we are doesn't fit any more. This old myth of humanity has been so thoroughly institutionalized with so much written about it, based upon the various versions of the myth in many cultures. Many professions are based on its mystery; and many innocent young people have died for it, that it has become a fact of life in many people's minds that are not open for discussion. However, the old myth is giving way as a natural course of events to a new myth based upon new discoveries in psychology, along with modern medical research and its discoveries.

The old myth temporarily solved the mystery of human nature by looking outward toward another mysterious world, the unreachable unknowable heavens, for centuries. Since space travel, and sensory confirmation, that heavenly place of rest has been brought into serious question.

A new myth has been offered by clinical experience and medical science, this time looking for answers to the mysteries of human nature toward the inner world of the human body. This sensory conformation is made possible through the use of psychology, of electro-chemistry, gene patterns, modern research techniques, scientific instrumentation and, human intuition. As the result of this research effort, the story qualifies as a myth, since there are still many more unknowns—mysteries of human nature—to be examined.

The change of myth for the individual involves a change of images of the human Self. The image of the old myth is a person with one brain with a single central nervous system, which requires an external source of control to manage the duality of its personality—the Self with a dual personality of good and evil. The new image of the individual involves two sources of intelligence, the upper brain with its central nervous system (CNS), and a second brain with its separate nervous system in the gut, the enteric nervous system (ENS). This second intelligence center provides the inner source of organismic self-control when properly nourished throughout the growth process. The mystery of this second center of intelligence, involves the DNA/RNA, installed at conception, and entered into every cell as the new organism develops. Our studies have shown that the concept of good and evil disappears from the image, while Self Control and Self Acceptance takes its place when the inner needs of the organism are fulfilled. When cultural attention is directed toward a full life for each child in his and her early learning experience, there should be far less concern for his future behavior as an adult.

The new image includes the fact that the second center of intelligence is installed during the development of the fetus and is completed and operating at birth. While only the neurons for potential neuro-sensory growth of the CNS are available at birth, the intelligence of the upper brain is dependent on the post-birth development of the externally directed sensory skills (sight, sound, taste, touch, and smell are dependent upon the quality or the environments to which the newborn is exposed). Thus, the upper brain cavity is essentially empty at birth and fills as experience is obtained, as Dr Lise Eliot points out, on a "first come first served" basis-pretty much "the luck of the draw." [2]

Because of these temporal differences in the development of the human organism—the second brain first and the upper brain last—we postulate that what Dr. Gershon calls *the second brain*,[3] the gut brain, contains the stabilizing influence—the feed back of its wisdom gathered over eons of time (and of the two brains, it is the most likely link to archetypal human history) and the wisdom of its stability, its experience maintaining the species. Thus, this feedback becomes the built-in direction toward the organism's destiny.

Under normal conditions, the two centers of intelligence work in harmony together sending signals of conditions in each other's domain. The sensory signals are normally strong and multiple while the signals from the inner gut are feeling and are easily overwhelmed by the senses, and easily ignored without special attention. It is this special attention we seem not to have learned or are loosing, which seems to be the cause of the communications disconnect between the two centers, and this deprives us of our needed directions and causes us to experience an unhealthy amount of stress symptoms.

Under conditions of stress, the gut brain can become a disturbing influence to the upper, externally directed brain. When the outside environment fails to meet the needs of the organism, or the upper brain attempts to distort the directions from the second brain, depending on the degree of stress, the inner second brain can reduce the energy available to the organism, thereby causing it to reconsider. There seems to be a constant dialog between the two brains at all times. This constant feed-back produces an interesting set of regulating qualities of behavior and suggest that it is the possible sources of ethics, morality, and the boundary conditions of Acceptance and Control of the Self and of others, and of other forms of life—*A Reverence For Life*, as described by Albert Schweitzer in the last century published in the periodical Christendom. (1 [1936]: 225-39).

THE NEW FUNCTIONAL IMAGE OF HUMANITY

If we take time to reflect on the inner awareness of our own human decision-making process, we find the presence of arguments or discussions, which are now, or have been known to be in process internally, "Should I or shouldn't I buy that dress…that new PC…that new car? Or, should I buy the double-decker with cheese and mayo or just with lettuce and tomato? Shall I kiss her or will that ruin our relationship? Shall I come out with truth or should I wait to see if anyone discovers the lie?" This always so simple internal dialogue goes on with the result that we can hopefully and finally make up our minds. The sensory input (sight, sound, taste, touch smell) can momentarily pull us away from ourselves, and our awareness of inner need pulls us back. It is the internal feedback, which cautions the want (seeing, hearing, touching tasting, smelling), which drives the desire back to the inner voice of necessity.

From these simple examples, we can intuit the functional use of two centers of intelligence in decisions of a far more serious nature. We can intuit the value to the individual of a more conscious awareness of the limitations and benefits of the outward attraction of the senses for curiosity, risk, and change, along with the value of a more conscious awareness of inward attention to gut feelings for structure, stability, and safety. One moment we may need energy for Control and the next moment we may need energy for Acceptance. Without the awareness of internal feedback, we seek the need for control and acceptance from outside sources. There is nothing new about this new image except the awareness that we have built-in structures available to us internally to help make healthy and sometimes disruptive choices in our lives. Upon studying this built-in structure, it becomes clear that we all need to be more conscious of and experienced with the inner requirements of human nature, both individually and collectively. Is humanity ready to use our intuition to explore what a new image opens for us—the conscious awareness of inner human needs in making healthy choices? If so, we will find human need is an undeniable force of nature with which to be reckoned, as we examine both individual and collective decision-making.

The Image we have painted requires substance and attention to make it work—it has inner needs. In the past, traditional thought has tended to view these so-called, sub-conscious needs of less importance than external needs like food, water, shelter, mobility, and our senses, sight, sound, taste, touch, and smell. Not that we can't do without any one of them, some combinations of them, or a temporary loss of them, but we consider any loss of them puts us at a social disadvantage to compete in the outside world. In such a situation, we are offered a handicap for our limited ability to compete. It seems that this constitutes the cognitive results of our present view of human nature. With such a view of ourselves, we are aware of most of our external needs but hardly consider there are needs beyond the above that require cognitive attention to the inside, where the vital processes are taking place—even when cognition sleeps. We tend to take the inner needs for granted until some unusual feeling occurs, or something goes wrong internally and we are suddenly hungry, thirsty, need to urinate, need to defecate, we can't breathe, we can't eat, we can't sleep, or we feel unusual pain. It is the unusual feeling that now gets our attention to the inner feelings—feelings that are the voice of internal intelligence. In our new human image, we have 'bundled' these external and inner necessities into the vital need for Attention, which is experienced as a feeling of Acceptance.

The other inner necessity of human nature, which brings the need for Acceptance into balance, is the need to be in charge of our own space and time, our own lives. If not freely given, nature provides the energy and the will to take Control, or die for that natural right. The Control side of balanced necessity with Acceptance, provides human nature with the learned possibility of caring for others personal and social lives. We have a simple way of explaining this necessity of this balance: If you take too much Control in human relationships, others may loose interest in you and pay less Attention. If you give others too much Attention, others may take over and Control your life. The dynamics of this duality reflects the constant struggle for a delicate balance of these two organic needs.

We believe this balance is a learned skill, best learned as soon as possible after birth in an environment of the home and preschool, and nourished for the rest of school-life. We think this early learning process will be a key, which can unlock doors to many stubborn social problems, but will take a long time to develop and install in a public education system.

The human needs, to which we refer in our writing, are the inner needs that support neurological-pathway development, which define the species, in addition to the food, air, water, and light, required for all life. Since these needs are so closely tied to both nervous systems and were expressed by all individuals who seriously participated in the Somatic Reflection Process (SRP) with us throughout our years of counseling, we postulated that these inner needs were instinctual needs and were possibly possessed by most if not all of the animal kingdom. If we look for a valid reason to support the declaration of the "instinctual needs" of Control and Acceptance, we might look for that which the adult animal is willing to risk its life—that for which it would be willing to die? We might also look at the natural behavior of a newborn for a need of direct development of Self Control and Self Acceptance. Perhaps we might help validate these essential needs in its post birth choices, and even in the pre-natal order of development, for in that process there may be clues.

It also seems reasonable to accept the idea that our ancestors climbed down out of the trees, spending more time on the ground, risking their lives to improve their Freedom to find the Acceptance of a possible mate. Countless numbers of people have offered to die for the cause of Freedom—Self

Control, and the protection of their loved one's special Acceptance. Many have made the offer of their lives to defend their country so that their Freedom and Acceptance would improve. Some lived to come home to find no more Freedom or no more Acceptance than they had the day they enlisted. Since it was a life or death decision for them, it is likely that at some point in their lives, the inner force of nature will well up inside them and explode. Sadly, it is then that rank, metals, and names like "Hero" cannot equate with and balance out the physical and mental damage the decisions that were made have done in their lives.

As we have pointed out, Dr Michael Gershon now defines the image of the human being with two centers of intelligence—the ENS and the CNS—in a medical breakthrough. The plan for the ENS (Enteric Nervous System), given to the future zygote at conception by its parents, contains a portion of animal history, which provides the zygote with plans to form its basic animal characteristics. That plan must contain the electro-chemical knowledge to produce all necessary materials to complete the job on site by birth-time. It must have the voice of feeling to communicate its importance to the cognitive domain, and take the responsibility for producing energy for the entire animal at birth. For the CNS (Central Nervous System), it must learn what is in the best interest of the organism at all times and constantly communicate what it sees, hears, tastes, touches, and smells of the environments in the outside world—its domain. It must recognize and gather the fuel to feed the digestive system, learn and remember through experience what not to feed it. It must learn to recognize many forms of danger and remember how to avoid them through experience. The CNS must learn how to communicate and deal with other animals in diverse environments outside, as well as, the language of critical feeling with the ENS inside. And finally, the CNS must learn to integrate all the information it has received from the outside world with the information from the ENS inside, and be prepared to function for the benefit and welfare of the individual organism, at millisecond speed—lots of room for mistakes.

If we reflect for a moment on the images we carry of all other humans in our environments, all of us will have the same basic idea of a range of behavior we might experience from everyone we meet. We will find the same basic operating system—much like the basic operating system of a computer. What will be different will be the 'software' we have acquired from our individual environmental experiences—that which has been added and stored from the individual experience we might call the personality. This stored information, the impact of individual's experiences, we will never know about each other until each chooses to share it or until we show enough interest in each other to deserve it.

The simple answer to the question, "why is this potentially disturbing functional separation of the two systems necessary?" The answer seems to be in the fact that the two systems are designed to do two different jobs, and the feedback, which this separation of function provides, stabilizes the function of the whole organism. Dr. Gershon expresses functional feed back in this manner: "In contrast to the remainder of the peripheral nervous system [central nervous system], however, the enteric nervous system [the internal intelligence] does not necessarily follow commands it receives from the [upper] brain or spinal cord; nor does it inevitably send the information it receives back to them. The enteric nervous system can, when it chooses, process data its sensory receptors pick up all by themselves, and it can act on the basis of those data to activate a set of effectors that it alone controls. The enteric nervous system is thus not a slave of the body. It is a rebel, the only element of the peripheral nervous system that can elect not to do the bidding of the [upper] brain or spinal cord." [4]

This use of feedback allows the system to be self-correcting when the need arises, which is probably a major reason why this dual system of thinking and feeling has been so successful. The presence of an ancient brain in the skull, with the attached intelligence of the enteric nervous system in the belly, has its neuron circuits scattered throughout the entire organism before birth. This arrangement seems to provide quality control for the development of the main brain, which nestles around the ancient brain, as it develops after birth. The main brain seems to be directed to fill in the empty space as it develops its function to cope with the external environments, as does the connected central nervous system fill in the body space as it develops. Not only are the two connected brains in intimate space in the skull, but also the nerve cells of each system are intertwined in the organism's physical space where there is a need for combined cooperation between the two systems. Otherwise, one system would operate without external steerage—the ENS—and the CNS would operate without effective energy; and there would no feedback for corrective action. Such systems would probably eliminate the intuitive possibility of the organism. Like the computer, the efficiency of the system would be lost, and the organism as we know it, would probably have been extinct ages ago. [5]

The conclusion, that the structure of the human nervous systems stabilize each other with self–correcting feedback, gives us pause to wonder why we have so much trust in the dependability of human intuitive intelligence when we relate to things, and so much distrust for that same human intelligence when we apply the model to human social issues? We could consciously be using the dependability of the human nervous systems as an analogue for ethics and morality instead of an analogue for depravation, as we now tend to use it. There seems to be much more intelligence involved in the learning process than most of us ever imagined. And, there is so much more importance to be assigned to the cognitive awareness of these human faculties in educational foundations, parental and teacher training, and educational environments, in the early years of life, than many of us have ever consciously defined.

QUESTIONING HUMAN NATURE AND THE GUT DECISION

We had a colleague recently ask us how we can see human nature as essentially good with all the history of wars we seem to keep moving through as an entire humanity. Of course, we can see why people would question the idea that we have caring natures, for that is hardly observable when we focus on the amount of wars and greed we see in this modern world, and in our entire human history, at least up until now. From looking at our behavior alone, humanity may even appear the opposite of caring and seem to have a propensity, at least in part, toward conflict and destruction. But upon careful examination, we find that it is often our misguided or misinformed thinking process that gets us into wars and conflicts, and it is our guts that signal us to be caring and peaceful and to care about human needs.

It is certainly true that we have a choice to either become more conscious and follow our instinctual nature or become less conscious of it and follow an external set of principles. And under the stress of survival or responsibility we are often observed following a dogma or set of ill-conceived principles we accept from an external authority. This outside source of thought could even be a well-meaning parent or mentor that does not take into account our instinctual needs as human beings with their judgments of what would be a wise course to follow. We may even go so far as to think we are following a gut feeling in a decision to wage and participate in something as destructive as war or some other violence. And we may even proclaim that we are following our gut and are "Gut Men or Gut Women", when all the while we are unconsciously and mistakenly following our convoluted thinking based on someone else's opinion of what is right and wrong for us to do. Our only gut decision may be, in that case, not to stand alone from our external authorities in our decision-making process and thus we willingly give up the freedom of being a true decider of a difficult question in our lives to gain some feeling of acceptance.

But then this confusion of whether we have really followed our thinking or gut feelings or a combination of both is understandable because there is no consensus on what our gut feelings and instinctual needs as human beings are, or if we even have them beyond biological responses attached to biological needs of food consumption. It may seem like a bold statement to say that any logical life principles we follow that do not take into account ones need for both acceptance from other human beings and the freedom to respond naturally (and thus feel in control of ones own life responses), will fail us. And if we follow these external, unnatural principles, we take the risk of our behavior running us into walls and fighting windmills in the air that make us appear to the external world as instinctually destructively driven and untrustworthy. When in truth, no one is destructively driven from an instinctual gut level, nor is any one intrinsically built to need conflict or war, not for growth or we should say particularly not for growth and attainment of the feeling of fulfilling one's purpose in life. And surely creativity does not need conflict as it flourishes during truly nurturing periods in both our personal and collective history.

This leads us to the question of our future and what it will be like when we as a humanity are, in our evolved future selves, consciously in touch with our gut instinctual feelings and we accept the new image of human nature.

I bring to you a mirror new—a glass of introspection clear,
That illusion shows, and sooty fear that spots thy mind.
Thou wilt also find this mirror new would loyal show, all
true, The "Inner You" that's veiled in flesh
and never doth appear.
(Paramahansa Yogananda, 1983, p. 156)

CHAPTER FIVE:

THE DEVELOPMENT OF THE SOMATIC REFLECTION PROCESS AND A NEW SCHOOL OF GUT PSYCHOLOGY

The principles discussed in this chapter were developed, recorded, and based on our counseling experiences that we carried out in the 1970s, prior to the neurobiological discoveries of gut intelligence by Dr. Michael Gershon[1] and other supporting modern neurological research, which we will discuss in a later chapter. We offer it here as a clear discussion of how these clinical studies demonstrated the relationship of the two separate organic systems of brain and gut, and how they can function for optimal emotional health and creativity of the person in an educational setting. We conducted these clinical studies during a five-year period as career counselors with hundreds of community college students, of a variety of ages and nationalities, with both genders. The following account of our clinical studies demonstrates the need for conscious attention to the awareness of the gut area in the educational process of people if they are to learn to make healthy life choices for themselves and others.

This chapter provides a background in modern psychological accepted thought and research by many of the founders of psychology, and then makes the connection of the question of how the Somatic Awareness Process (SRP) is a natural evolution of Depth Psychology or Analytical Psychology, including Somatic Psychology, Humanistic Psychology, Individual Psychology, Nondual Psychotherapy, and Object Relations, combined together and brought forward to meet the modern human psyche and nature. We first discuss the principles of the theoretical model of the psyche that underlie the Somatic Reflection Process and then demonstrate how these principles are grounded in the works of Depth Psychology.

We have expanded our original understanding of these principles to include a more complete awareness of a Jungian prospective. These principles are sources of discovery and arise in questions rather than answers. The underlying principles that we are presenting were found by examining how we developed our work and the mysteries that intrigued us and led us to develop a strategy or technique for working with others.

FINDING THE SOURCE OF INNER CONFLICT AND STRESS

Many of the people who came to us for career counseling indicated that they were confused about what they wanted to do for a career. Either they had no idea of what they wanted to do for an occupation, or they felt a conflict between what they thought they should do and what they felt they wanted to do. Many people did not know how to make a career life decision because they lacked awareness of what was intrinsically valuable to them. People expressed an inner conflict between what they thought and what they felt, which often resulted in an emotional crisis and a deep feeling of emptiness.

To help people with this inner conflict, we first turned the father of analytical psychology Dr. Carl Jung's[2] theory of typology to explore the difference in thinking and feeling. Jung posits that there are two distinct rational functions of judgment of the psyche—thinking and feeling. Thinking and feeling are grouped together as ways a person makes judgments and decisions. Jung defines the thinking function as bringing "given presentations into conceptual connection".[3] He defines the use of the thinking function as the way a person conceptualizes experiences with the world using rationality and logic. Jung defines the feeling function as "a process that takes place between the ego and a given content ... that imparts to the content a definite value in the sense of acceptance or rejection".[4] The feeling function relates to what a person values and to the question of acceptance or rejection of experience.

Dr. Jung views both functions as rational because they are "founded upon reasoning, judging functions".[5] In his theory of types, he points out the problems of being one-sided concerning the dominance of one of these functions. Jung speaks of the one-sided dominance of thinking as happening when the feeling function becomes dependent upon thinking. In this case, feeling is merely kept as an accompaniment to thinking. In some cases of extraverts, the thinking function may learn to operate around external systems of thought that conflict with the feeling function. Thus, the person's thinking may not be relevant to what is valued internally and is divorced from the awareness of the body. In this case, thinking dominates and the feeling function is suppressed. Likewise, the feeling function may be so dominant and one-sided in a person's awareness that it overrides any possibility of further thinking about a situation or circumstance. Dr. Jung considered neither case to be an example of balanced reasoning judgment. Many people we were seeing were suffering from the domination of their thinking function and expressed the emptiness that domination caused.

Dr. Donald Winnicott,[6] who was a British pediatrician and psychoanalyst and influenced the field of Object Relations theory, suggests that the origin of the dominance of externalized thinking begins in early childhood. He found that the child creates a *false self*, hiding the authentic self or true inner being. This happens because the caregiver did not mirror the child's authentic gestures; rather the infant was forced to comply with the caregiver's gestures. This results in the formation of the false self. This false self is only able to decide what it needs in relation to the values of others. The child learns the necessity of dominating inner needs and feelings by pleasing others.

Combining the theories of Dr. Jung and Dr. Winnicott pointed us to the understanding that the conflict our clients were having was between their thinking and emotional feelings and that it actually began in early childhood with a loss of awareness of their inner needs. Our task was then to develop a process that would assist people in recovering the awareness of their inner needs and bringing that awareness into the decision making process in the present issues of their lives. This opened up the question of whether there is a record in the psyche of how well these inner needs are met. Was there a stored memory of the consciousness of these inner needs as they were lived and met or not met? If so, how could we access this record?

Certainly this record would not be accessed exclusively through the use of the thinking function, for it was the thinking that dominated the feelings and inner needs in the first place. We ruled out the idea of merely thinking back to early childhood recollections to find when a person first lost the awareness of having inner needs. We realized that our explorations must include emotional and somatic feelings, as a guide to access inner needs. But where were the feelings located, which ones should we use, and how would we go about using them to find this record of feeling experiences and inner needs?

THE MBTI AND THE DEVELOPMENT OF THE SOMATIC REFLECTION PROCESS

Early on, when we began our work at SFCC in Career Gap, we began to enjoy a special working relationship with Dr. Mary McCauley, Director, University of Florida's Typology Lab, and our meetings with Isabel Myers and Dr. Mary McCauley, on the Myers-Briggs Type Indicator (MBTI). We mention the importance of the MBTI in our work because it was through interpreting our own results before using it as part of a battery of tests in the Career Gap Center that we first had a need to reflect on our early childhood experience to assess if our type results had changed as adults, and if so, what that might have meant in serving our needs as a person. We were in search of the understanding if our type results were true for us naturally or if our type had changed due to necessity and environmental adaptation. And if our type had changed, we were interested to understand if the early type was more satisfying of our human needs. This deep unconscious information could only be accessed through a reflection on our feelings, rather than our thinking process, beginning in childhood and brushing up to the present time. And it was in our personal exploration and validation of the results of the MBTI that the Somatic Reflection Process had its beginning and served as a further guide toward understanding a new image of human nature.

The MBTI was central to the development of our career counseling and professional work in the 1970s with the enteric nervous system, the instinctual gut response. The MBTI gave us an inclusive view of personality, which we could share with clients in our career guidance, and it provided a model of how people perceive and make judgments in life and why they prefer some types of experiences instead of other types. The model of typology was very useful in helping people enhance decision-making toward positive experiences in career and life in general. At the same time, using the MBTI model caused us the need to find a way to validate the findings, which the inventory results presented. We soon realized people needed, just as we ourselves had found with our own type results, to reflect on the very early years of their lives up to the present in order to find for themselves if their type results were always true or had changed over the years due to environmental pressures, and to find what the results meant for each person individually. The MBTI provided an initial logical model for us to assist the person to discover their feeling experiences. This model was both useful to people and understandable. It was a positive rather than an exclusive view of what was considered good or bad, as other personality inventories available at that time seemed to represent.

Many people in America during this post '60s period were going through profound transformations in their lives and experiencing confusion as they attempted to make drastic changes in career and life style toward the goal of higher personal fulfillment. We soon found the majority of people coming into the center not only had absolutely no idea of a suitable career direction for them but also had no idea who they were inside. We found that the usual career interest tests were meaningless for these people because they had no real idea of their own inner feelings and thus had no way to determine if the results were accurate and thus useful. Often the test-results would point the person in a direction that had more to do with their cultural and family values than their true inner feelings, instincts, and personal values.

Fortunately, the Myers-Briggs Type Indicator (MBTI) was at this time, in the mid '70s, being extensively researched at the Type Lab by Dr. Mary McCauley at the University of Florida, so we had the opportunity to abandon our idea of using standard personality tests for career counseling and employ the MBTI. For several years we had the opportunity to administer, interpret, and gather data from the MBTI for hundreds of people using the services of Career Gap and fed this data to the University of Florida Typology Lab, headed by Dr. Mary McCauley. Because of this association with Dr. McCauley, we were introduced to Mrs. Briggs-Myers and had a number of private meetings with both of them.

Isabel Myers would come to town several times a year to check on how the research was going at the Type Lab. The MBTI was used at that time, more locally at the University of Florida and, perhaps, a few other university communities. Dr. McCauley and Mrs. Briggs-Myers were struggling to provide additional research data on the use of the MBTI, though its validity and reliability had been proven in the early '60s. But the funding was so skimpy for the research project that we had to meet at Dr. McCauley's home, because the Type Lab at the university was just a small office where she had a computer and one part-time assistant, whose name, our memories have barely recorded was Penny. (We can now actually remember more about her personality type than her name, as she was a very friendly ENFP). Funding was a struggle and on several occasions Dr. McCauley was not sure if they would be able to keep the Lab open due to the lack of support. But somehow they managed to continue their work, even with occasional cutbacks. Perhaps it was as they thought and on occasion told us, that their intuitive preferences, both being INFP's, kept them persistently focused in moving forward, despite financial lack of funds, toward a vision of a future time when their research would be accepted and fully funded (Personal communication with Dr. McCauley and Mrs. Isabel Briggs-Myers, 1975).

On one occasion during a meeting in which we were handing over data to Dr. McCauley for their research, and Isabel Myers was also visiting, we asked Isabel if she would come talk to one of our freshman classes, an introductory course in psychology (BE100), in which we were using the MBTI. She graciously accepted and appeared the next week. It was long before the days of cell phones, and there was not an easy way to affirm the appointment, so we were a bit surprised and very much elated that she actually came. When she arrived at the class, she was wearing a simple housedress and had her hair in a bun. She was a lady in her early 70's and made no pretense of being a professional. She sat with her legs crossed, in front of the students, her hands folded in her lap, and a relaxed sweet smile on her face. Everyone seemed to accept her as Grandmother for the evening imparting the knowledge of a wise old woman. The following is an account of what we remember of Isabel Myers' personal communication to the class (Personal communication 1975):

> *My Mother, Catherine Briggs, was a woman that noticed even small things about people. She wasn't a psychologist and I don't think she had read a word of Carl Jung. She just noticed the different relatives acted the opposite from each other when they all got together for Thanksgiving dinner. She would say, Uncle [Hank] always talks about only facts and Aunt [Sarah] always talks about possibilities. Sometimes they had whole conversations, my mother would say, without really listening to each other. She wouldn't judge any one for being so different. She was just*

interested that it seemed to be that way. So she sat down over a period of time and wrote all the characteristics of each relative and made up a questionnaire. It was very different from the one you take now, although it asked about the same basic kinds of preferences.

Isabel Myers went on to tell the story of how the MBTI was developed, and we remember her saying she helped her mother by working with a Jungian psychologist to develop the inventory, fitting Jungian theory. What was really interesting to us was her account of how the Myers Briggs Type Indicator had its root beginnings as a homespun personal inventory. It was born out of the keen observations of the every day experiences with people of Catherine Briggs and her interest in helping people communicate with each other with greater understanding.

Most of the discussions we had in our meetings with Isabel Myers and Dr. McCauley centered around accounts of the research in the Type Lab. They were both quite excited that the research was going so well and the findings were coming up significant for certain job categories. They found it interesting that elementary school teachers came out a majority of sensing types and college teachers were showing results of being a majority of intuitive types. We talked about the implications of how type affects learning styles and how the difference in type can explain intuitive types who may do better in higher math like algebra while having had difficulty adding and subtracting, and sensing types doing well in applied math areas of study as a career choice. They also found a the difference between the type outcome of police professionals—being sensing, types, and the university students—being intuitive types, and mused over ways they could bridge the communication gap between these two types during student protests that were quite prevalent on campus at this time in the '70s.

Over and over, Dr McCauley and Mrs. Myers expressed that we all have the ability to understand each other and thus communicate more effectively if we could understand our different preferences in type. We do not think it was Jung's intention that we label ourselves and obsess about our category or label or type. And we think that the MBTI was meant to be used by both Isabel Myers and Katherine Briggs as simply a way of thinking about ourselves and our gifts, not a device to trick us into a typology box in our minds, but as a tool to guide us in life decision-making and communication with others. We base our opinion on the many talks we had personally with Isabel Myers and her close colleague, Dr. Mary McCauley, whose explanations of typology were always flexible and open to the person's inner decision about himself or herself. We will add that both Isabel Myers, her mother Katherine Briggs, and Dr. McCauley were all Introvert Intuitive Feeling Perceptive (INFP) types, according to what we were told in our conversations with Dr McCauley and Isabel Myers. True to their types, they meant the MBTI to be a flexible and perceptive tool that the person could use as a guide to illuminate one's inner experiences and accept their unique gifts of perception and judgment.[6]

READING LIFE BACKWARDS

It was clear to us as counselors that the MBTI was a useful tool for people because it provided a structure with which to use in sorting out who we are and what our preferences are in viewing and experiencing the world. And it was clear that we would need to reflect back in time in order to discover the authentic feeling responses and the authentic type preference of the person.

As we view our lives beginning in the present time and read the backwards in time, we see an aspect of our being that does not relate to the development and environment we have experienced but rather to an innate aspect of our being. Dr. James Hillman says this when he posits that "reading life backwards enables you to see how early obsessions are the sketchy performances of behaviors now".[8] It is from this reading of our lives backwards in time that we experience a sense of the timelessness of our inner being. A door then can open to us to view an essence within ourselves that has always been there as the inner truth of our being and is continuing to live in us in the present. It is as if we are "looking in the mirror"[9] of our lives as we engage in reading life backwards and see the original image of the essence of our being.

We are accustomed to looking in a forward fashion, a progression from early life to the present, to tell the story of our lives in a linear sequence of events that emphasizes a left-brain causal view of who we have been and what situations and details has had an effect upon who we are today. However, Dr. Hillman demonstrates that we can only find our true inner essence through a right brain, acausal (rather than causal) view of our lives in which we become aware of a part of ourselves that has always been within us. He emphasizes the importance of breaking through the fixed idea in psychotherapy today that we are who we are in the present moment primarily because of our past experiences. Instead, he suggests that through reading life backwards we find that we are today who we are because of a spirit, or daemon, that has always been within us, guiding us toward the fulfillment of our life's calling, the natural design of in our very DNA.

But upon what within ourselves do we reflect backwards to view this "mirror of our lives"[10] that Dr. Hillman has spoken of so eloquently? Upon what do we reflect to find the most inner being that we are? Is there a signal within us that can lead us on the path to become conscious of our true inner being so that we might direct our lives from this inner reference? And if we became aware of our inner being, what would we find is the true essence of our inner being? How would we then define what it means to be a human being with a human nature? Would we find that our inner nature is aggressive and uncaring of other members of the human family? Are we doomed to stay in conflict through wars and aggression due to inheriting an inner nature that does not care about other human beings and must be controlled by a rigid code of morality? Or is it possible that the human nature each of us has inherited cares about life other than our own? Perhaps we would find that the wars and aggression of humankind throughout history have happened because we have not followed our nature. Could our aggression and wars be attributed to our lack of consciousness of our nature rather than our nature itself? Could reflection upon our inner nature lead us to a heightened consciousness that would direct our humanity away from aggression and war toward unity and peace?

These are the pressing questions that led us initially to explore our own inner nature and to discover a process of reflection on somatic feelings for finding the center of our beings.

THE FEELING OF EMPTINESS AND FULLNESS IN THE GUT

The more we worked in career counseling with people who felt confused as to what they really wanted to do, the more it became clear to us that the problem was not in their feeling responses but in their way of thinking and viewing themselves. We found that a person's thinking could be borrowed from someone else's thinking, but the somatic feeling responses between the hara region (the area directly below the stomach) and the solar plexus (the area where the lowest ribs conjoin at the breast bone) were connected to more instinctual needs. Through our own reflections and reflections with hundreds of other people, we found that these somatic feeling responses consistently served the state of the organism itself. We posited from our experience that these somatic feelings were a reliable center of reference reflecting the basic instinctual needs of the person.

We found in our counseling work that it was important for life decisions to be made with the person's somatic feeling responses as a fact considered in the premise of their logic. If the premise of the thinking process does not consider a person's own genuine needs, the conclusions that are derived from that premise are irrelevant to the organism's needs. Not only are the conclusions irrelevant to the inner needs of the person, but also we found with both ourselves and our clients that a feeling of a split between body and mind occurred. This split was caused by the body following an internal reference (the somatic feeling response) and the mind following an external reference (a view borrowing someone else's perspective). On the other hand, if the premise of logical thinking takes into account the instinctual needs of the person, then the conclusion drawn is directed towards fulfilling these needs, and the organism can take full responsibility for its feelings.

Because many people expressed to us a deep sense of emptiness, we sought to explore this feeling. Object Relations and Self Psychologists point to emptiness as the common feeling that people attach to the lack of expression of their inner needs. Without mirroring from others there is a lack of development of the authentic sense of self, and people often feel emptiness.[11] This lack of development of the authentic self often is based on learning a way of thinking that is compliant with people external to the person rather than the person's own inner feelings and values. We postulated that if a person was overly dominated by acculturated thinking that suppressed the awareness of feeling values and emotions, the organism suffered because the person's inner needs were not met. The emotions seemed to be the link between the body and the mind. Emotional feelings were sensed in the body and thinking was experienced in the mind. If emotional feelings were suppressed, pushed out of one's thinking awareness, decisions and behavior were made that did not take into account the personal state of the organism. This lack of inner needs being met resulted in a profound feeling of emptiness and lack of meaning in the person's life. Having a sense of meaning seemed to be defined by the people coming to see us as the experience of feeling they were moving toward fulfilling their inner needs and purpose. Having a sense of lack of meaning in life seemed to be defined as the experience of people feeling they were not moving toward fulfilling their inner needs and purpose.

Dr. Carl Jung[12] in his description of the conflict of the ego with its two contrary tendencies toward independence and the feeling of belongingness speaks to the feelings that result from the lack of experiencing meaning and inner needs. The persona and the shadow are a pair of opposites that stand in the ego as polarities. The persona is the mask we show the world designed to make impressions upon others as well as to "conceal the true nature of the individual".[13] This *public personality*[14] facilitates adaptation to the demands of the society in which the person lives. It functions in the personal consciousness and could be described as the "protective skin on the body of the psyche or the face that is presented to the world in order to facilitate adaptation"[15]. It is exclusively centered on its relation to the objective world.

While wearing this mask may bring about adaptation and social acceptance, it may not serve the inner needs of the person. The shadow contains repressed material from consciousness, including the tendencies that conflict with the persona and are deemed negative. Dr. John Conger,[16] eminent depth psychoanalysts, and a bioenergetics trainer and founder of Analytic Somatic Therapy (AST), points to the body as the container for the shadow content. We could see a relationship to this repression of material and the emotions such as what we call fear, guilt, and hostility. Emotions like fear, guilt and hostility may arise when there is a conflict in the ego between what is rooted in the persona that moves us to adapt to the objective world, and what is rooted in the shadow that emerges as an urge to gain independence or a feeling of control of one's own responses to life.

We found that as people talked to us about the confusion that they experienced, they often expressed the emotion of guilt, which they generally described feeling somewhere in the solar plexus to the heart area of the body. Many people also described this feeling of guilt as being accompanied by an underlying feeling of emptiness in the hara (the area just below the navel) to the solar plexus (the area where the lowest ribs conjoin at the breast bone). In exploring this emptiness related to the emotion of guilt, people expressed that it was due to the lack of the feeling of acceptance and was accompanied by a strong sense of aloneness. This is understandable if we look at developmental psychopathologist Dr. Robert Weis's statement that loneliness appears to be coming from the emotional isolation of hiding our authentic selves from others. "The sense of utter aloneness may be phrased in terms of an empty inner world, in which case the individual may say that he or she feels empty, dead, or hollow".[17] We postulated that underlying the emotion of guilt, there is a deep feeling of emptiness in the gut region of the body that often identifies the lack of fulfillment of the person's need for acceptance.

If people are too identified with their persona, they may over adapt to the desires of the social world and lose an awareness of the inner identity of the personality.[18] In this dilemma, Dr. David Winnicott[19] found that the person experiences the false self and loses awareness of the authentic self. We found that people often expressed a feeling of fear of what it might be like if their authentic self was ever disclosed to others. Also, they expressed feeling out of control because the shadow aspects of themselves had to be suppressed in order to be acceptable to others. We found that underlying the emotion of fear, people often expressed a deep feeling of emptiness in the gut area of the body. This emptiness went along with the awareness that they were unable to be their authentic selves. A feeling of loss of control occurred as a result of this lack of feeling free to express themselves. When people believed they had to play a role or over-identify with the persona, they felt a loss of freedom of the use and awareness of their own innate responses to life. We postulated that underlying the emotion of fear, there is a deep feeling of emptiness in the gut area of the body that often identifies the lack of fulfillment of the need for being in control of one's own response to life, that is, the lack of feeling free to respond naturally. We further postulated that if the meaning of experience of people's lives are set in meanings borrowed from outside authorities or in response to fulfilling the needs of others, there may be little experience of meaning and time spent toward fulfilling one's own inner needs.

While people expressed many emotional feelings related to what was happening in their objective world, the feeling of emptiness in their gut area seemed consistently to be more basic to the overall state of their organism. We postulated that the gut area response of emptiness and fullness is a gauge of whether the organism is getting what it needs in life or not—whether a person is on the path of being fulfilled in terms of innate needs and purpose, or is on the path of being empty and unfulfilled in terms of innate needs and purpose.

Often people expressed to us the lack of meaning in their lives as an emptiness felt in the pit of their stomachs. While they expressed many emotional feelings related to what was happening in their objective world, the feeling of emptiness in their gut area seemed consistently to be more basic to the overall state of their organism. Priest, academic theologian, and prolific author Matthew Fox[20] supports the awareness of this area of the body relating to the state of the organism. He draws upon Eastern thought that it is the source of the circulation of the essence of life energy. We postulated that the gut area response of emptiness and fullness is a gauge of whether the organism is getting what it needs in life or not—whether a person is on the path of being fulfilled in terms of innate needs and purpose or is on the path of being empty and unfulfilled in terms of innate needs and purpose.

The experience of emptiness in the gut is related to what Dr. Eugene Gendlin calls the *felt sense*,[21] the body's sense of a situation or event. Emptiness was not identified by the people we were seeing as having a conceptual aspect, as did emotions like guilt and fear. The awareness of emptiness was expressed as a purely somatic feeling without a logical cause or predicted outcome attached. While the felt sense is pre-conceptual, it holds the meaning of the inner experience. Emptiness in the gut area, like the felt sense, is not usually a sharp feeling like an emotion. In describing the felt sense, Dr. Gendlin points out that although an emotion might seem dominant at a given moment, "below it and behind it lie something huge and vague". [22] This hugeness and vagueness is not something that we experience by the mind but by the body. Emptiness was expressed to us as a general state of the organism that was felt in the body. Dr. Brian Wittine, Jungian analyst, posits that the body and psyche are distinct manifestations of the essential self, but not separate from it.

He points to the feeling of emptiness as an indication of this disconnection. "Being out of touch with the Self leaves us feeling unstable, empty, and ontologically insecure".[23] It is the body that is aware of our disconnection to our essential self and the body that feels the resulting stress.

The idea that there could be a felt sense like a gut feeling of emptiness or fullness underlying the emotional feelings, is reflected in theories of emotion that include an awareness of feedback from one's own body as contributing to the awareness of emotion. This is not to say that our emotions are based on our physical reactions alone. From the responses people were giving us in our counseling sessions, we postulated that the emotions are developed from the awareness of a combination of a person's perception of given situations and the feelings of emptiness or fullness experienced in the gut area. As the person begins to think about why the feeling in the gut is empty or full, emotions like guilt and fear are formed as a combination of thinking and feeling. "Because the thinking function could be influenced by the views of others, an emotional feeling could be a logical attempt to express the organismic state of being from an external rather than an internal view. This external view could be completely void of the awareness of the inner somatic, instinctual needs of the person and support a misinterpretation of the essence of the organism itself and its life purpose.

We found that these emotions, or psychosomatic feelings, were usually described by people as being experienced in the solar plexus to the heart area of the body; whereas, feelings of emptiness and fullness were described by people as being experienced in the hara to the solar plexus. We therefore postulated that there are two levels of feelings—emotional feelings and purely somatic instinctual feelings—with the solar plexus being the meeting point.

OUR INSTINCTUAL NEEDS

In reflecting upon our own feelings and facilitating the reflection process with our clients, we became aware that the two basic needs of acceptance and freedom-to-be-oneself were being constantly monitored by a feeling center in the gut area of the body. We found that the fulfillment of these needs was being registered as empty-full feelings. These feelings were experienced in the gut area of the body located between the hara and the solar plexus.

The lack of fulfillment of either the acceptance or freedom issues seemed to register as a feeling of emptiness; fulfillment of either issue seemed to register as a feeling of fullness. In order to understand how this occurs, as it may seem like an illogical equation, it is useful to imagine that our instinctual response center in the gut area is much like the gas gauge in a car. While empty and full are on extreme ends of the gauge, there seems to be fullness and emptiness that is relative to these extremes. If the gas gauge on a car is on empty and we pour into its tank even a gallon of gas, we can be elated in the fact that we can keep driving down the road, at least momentarily. We found that as long as people perceived that they were moving in the direction of gaining a balance of acceptance and freedom, they experienced a feeling of fullness, even though it may be *relative fullness*. Similarly, if people perceived that they were moving in the direction of a loss of a balance of these two basic needs, they experienced a feeling of emptiness, even though it may be *relative emptiness*. This relative degree of fullness and emptiness is implied when speaking of one's energy level in the common adage, "I'm running on empty." What people really mean by this is, "I'm running on a relative amount of emptiness, but I must also be relatively full or I could not move at all or even utter those words."

We found with ourselves and our clients that it is necessary to continually replenish one's experience of acceptance and freedom. They are vital needs and the emptiness and fullness that registers as a gauge of how well these needs are met, is engaged in the moment of experiencing. The somatic feelings in the hara area seem to reflect the sense of the moment. Just as eating a meal today registers a feeling of fullness that only lasts for a number of hours and we feel a need to eat again each day, the instinctual needs for acceptance and freedom are cyclic phenomena and require regular attention and maintenance to be fulfilled. For example, we may feel quite full if we already have acceptance and then, from some act of expressing the authentic self, begin to feel an additional sense of freedom. In this case, we may feel fullness with a balance of both needs for acceptance and freedom being met. This sense of fullness may be somewhat lasting, but the need to continue to take the freedom to respond naturally will surely become apparent with a growing feeling of emptiness if we repress our feelings and do not continue to experience freedom. Likewise, if we perceive a sudden loss of acceptance from important people in our lives, we could plummet with a growing feeling of emptiness and a condition of stress in the body.

We found that the basic needs for acceptance and freedom seemed to determine people's behavior. These two needs functioned much like a teeter-totter, with one need on each side of the scale. Often one need was given up for another, but the organism was constantly trying to find a balance of these two needs. We saw through reflection on feelings with our clients and ourselves that a struggle for a balance of these two needs was present in behavior from infancy throughout the entire span of adult life. We postulated that this urge to balance the two needs for acceptance and for freedom seems to be leading people toward the feeling of having fulfilled their unique purpose. Because these two needs were found consistently to be present in our clients, we viewed them as shared universally, and thus instinctual in the human family.

The duality and paradox of these two instinctual needs lies in the fact that there is really no such thing as acceptance without the freedom to be ourselves. People often would say I want to be loved for who I really am. And people found that when they were perfectly free, they desired most to share their experiences with someone else who would accept them as they truly are. Dr. David Viscott, who was a popular American psychiatrist that influenced the self-help approach using talk radio and syndicated TV along with the publication of a number of notable books, speaks to the importance of the fulfillment of both of these needs when he posits that the most fulfilling relationships are those in which people are free to be themselves. He views the feeling of loneliness in a relationship as the longing for the sacrificed part of oneself given up for the relationship. We postulated that it is essentially impossible to experience the essence of one instinctual need without the other.

Like the energy of yin and yang—opposites of light and dark forming a unity in our lives—or the Uroborous symbol —the completion of one world creating another in the natural evolution of the planet, we eternally seek a state of harmony and balance of our two instinctive human needs of acceptance and control, which are felt in our gut as emptiness and fullness. The urge for a balance of acceptance and freedom works in a similar fashion as does Dr. Jung's idea of the urge of the self-individuating through holding a union of opposites. We see in the natural world, or the holistic force of the morphic field described by biologist Rupert Sheldrake, this pattern of dual energies as opposites forming a unity, repeated again and again, and it is no surprise that our gut intelligence contains this same pattern originating, expressing, and evolving our human nature. We found in our counseling that if these needs do not feel like they exist in balance, it is as if they do not exist at all, and people feel empty. The people we counseled expressed that their lives were in constant transition, and that they were often experimenting and yearning for a state of harmony and balance of both acceptance and freedom of their own responses.

It became clear from the communication with people in our counseling experiences, that the instincts of the need for acceptance and for feeling free to respond naturally were rooted in the somatic experience. In our experience with people, the gauge for the fulfillment of both the instinctual needs of acceptance and freedom, like the biological need for food, was located in the gut area. The feelings of emptiness or fullness that were experienced as a signal of the instinctual needs of acceptance and freedom were easily confused with somatic feelings related to the biological instinct of hunger. With its attendant sensations of emptiness and fullness, this confusion concerning the similarity in feeling of these needs in the gut area seemed to explain why there was a propensity for some people toward over-consuming food. People expressed to us that they attempted to fill empty feelings in the gut area with food. This caused over-consumption and a denial of the real needs of the person that could result in food addictions, as well as other unhealthy life choices.

We found that in order to get in touch with their instinctual feeling responses, there was a need for people to reflect back to a much earlier time in their lives. The emotional issues in the present were generally what Dr. Jung identified as *triggers*[24] for issues that began in early childhood. It seemed sensible to trace the feelings in the present back to the earliest possible experience of that emotion so that the original source of the issue could be worked out. Reflecting on inner somatic feelings—on the impact of life and its meaning to the person—during earlier times gave people access to the record of their inner awareness. We often found that people were more aware of emotional feelings than the somatic instinctual feelings of emptiness and fullness. Because the emotional feelings are directly connected in the solar plexus, to the more purely somatic level of feelings in the hara, we used the awareness of them as a signal and starting point to become aware of the feelings of emptiness and fullness.

The process of reflection upon the somatic area of the hara and the solar plexus that we developed was designed to put people in touch with their instinctual responses. We found that the more experience people had reflecting on feelings, the more they became aware of a feeling of emptiness or fullness in this area of the body. These feelings of emptiness and fullness were experienced as a gauge of how well their instinctual needs were being met at any moment in their life. As we listened to the reports of our clients, we found that there were two universal instinctual needs that related to the feelings of emptiness and fullness— the need to be close to people with a feeling of acceptance; and the need to be free to express one's internal responses. The feeling of emptiness indicated that one or both of these needs were not being met, while the feeling of fullness indicated that the person was moving toward a balance of these needs being obtained. People expressed that the fulfillment of the need for both acceptance and freedom was an on-going process throughout their lives, from day to day, and from moment to moment.

While the need for acceptance and feeling connected to other human beings is more clearly understood, the need for freedom requires some clarification. The feeling of freedom was often expressed as feeling in control of one's own responses to life, rather than controlling one's responses to life and feeling out of control. Feeling in control was expressed as an internal, authentic, spontaneous, and natural experience of one's responses. Feeling out of control was expressed as complying with one's perceived external demands of the environment, both social and physical. This compliance was linked with a persistent control of one's responses. Paradoxically, this persistent control of one's responses was linked with feeling out of control. Consistently, people expressed that they experienced great effort in complying with what they imagined were the demands of others. In contrast to the experience of controlling oneself and feeling out of control, there was an effortlessness expressed in the experience of feeling in control and following one's natural responses.

In reflecting with people, we found that when the logical function of the ego became directly aware of the instinctive somatic feelings, the person felt a shift toward feeling full in the gut region of the body. Head, heart, and body became centered. This is similar to Dr. John Conger's idea of the beginning of individuation and the emerging from unconsciousness to consciousness through awareness of the solar plexus center to the heart center. He points out in *The Body as Shadow* that we remain stuck in our emotions if we remain blocked in our solar plexus center. The Somatic Reflection Process, a reflection on the feelings of emptiness and fullness in the gut area, was developed to accomplish the healing experience of unlocking the energy felt in this center. We postulated that for people to mend the body and mind split of consciousness, they must become aware of the feeling level of the gut area where the awareness of pure instinctual feeling without thinking is felt. It is then possible for the body and mind to make a link that mends the original split.

Reflecting on the instinctive somatic feelings of emptiness and fullness—on the impact of life and its meaning to the person—gave people access to the record of their inner awareness. People were often amazed to find that a reflection on the awareness of somatic feelings, rather than thinking back through the details of life events, gave them access to recover memories of both sensory information and the awareness of their inner instinctual needs. We found that when the logical function of the ego became directly aware of the instinctive somatic feelings of emptiness and fullness in the hara to the solar plexus, the person often experienced a reevaluation of the importance of their inner needs and a feeling shift occurred within them from an empty to a full feeling. The awareness of their instinctual needs often helped people to see the reasons for their behavior as children trying to fulfill these needs and to overcome the emptiness of not having them met. They often found in somatic reflection that the assessments they made as children about their behaviors were ones that they were told by authorities in their lives and were made with a child's limited information about the social and physical world. In the wisdom and light of adulthood, the new assessments of the reasons for their behavior were usually quite different from the ones they learned about themselves at the time of the early experience.

Dr. John Conger further suggests that an individual's center of consciousness can only be changed and refocused through body awareness, and that individuation is only possible through the awareness of the body. He posits that it is the unblocking of energy and the rising of awareness out of the manipura, or the solar plexus, into the anahata, or heart center, that begins the individuation process. He proposes that emerging from the manipura to the anahata is a psychic movement of energy from unconsciousness to consciousness of the self where thoughts and feelings are joined. It is not until we move the energy from the manipuri to the anahata that we can say our individuation process has really begun.

The third chakra of the body is located in the solar plexus starting just below the navel. It is considered the place where the essence of life and energy circulates in the body.[25]

According to Dr. Conger as long as our energy is blocked in the solar plexus, we are forever stuck in our emotions, with our feelings and thinking split off from each other. He further posits that with this split of body and mind, we can never find the vitality of our own center, nor can we fully experience the love and compassion for others of the heart center. This explains the importance of centering on the feelings in our solar plexus to unblock its energy flow.

With a profound new awareness of the essence of their inner being and human nature that was experienced in the Somatic Reflection Process, people expressed a feeling of compassion for themselves and others. This was followed by a release of tension in the body and a return of vital energy. With a greater feeling of self-acceptance, people indicated that they felt free again to be themselves and to make decisions about their lives. It was at this point that we found people began to experience a lack of confusion and a union of their thinking and feeling functions, consistently reported that they felt calm and centered with body and mind as one, and experienced a greater feeling of caring for themselves and others. People then expressed a feeling of a flow of creative energy and intuitive thought concerning what they wanted to do with their lives, and they were able to make career decisions and other personal choices that lead them toward healthy growth and development.

PRINCIPLES UNDERLYING THE TECHNIQUE OF THE SOMATIC REFLECTION PROCESS

In the following section, we include the principles that underlie the technique of the Somatic Reflection Process. We discuss the principles underlying the technique of centering on the feelings of unresolved issues, becoming conscious of our inner needs, and unblocking our emotions through the

Somatic Reflection Process. We also include a section on the principles of facilitating the Somatic Reflection Process.

Centering on the Feelings of Unresolved Issues

In an attempt to stay in the here and now, we developed the Somatic Reflection Process as a feeling process that emphasizes awareness in the body. It is important in this process for the person reflecting to hold the details of the experience in the mind, but to turn the awareness toward the inner experience of feelings in the body.

Such a reflection on the somatic instinctual feelings in the body, without the emphasis on the story or details of the life lived, is a reflection method that is the key to discovering for the first time the real meaning of experience. Both Jungian Analyst, teacher and author Dr. Marion Woodman as well as clinical psychologist and Depth Psychology dream work practitioner and author Dr. Jill Mellick stress the importance of listening to the body in order to get in touch with the deep cellular memory that it holds. We concurred their experience when we found in both our clinical studies and somatic reflection counseling that the stories and details may be helpful in understanding the environmental factors that the person is experiencing and the person's perceptions of the environment, but they are not memories stored in the body, nor arc they a part of the person. The details of stories are external to the person. Although these stories are in our memory, they are not the impact on a feeling level of the person's experience. We found that it is important to help the person discover the impact of the experience upon them within their body because that is what is still felt in the present. The impact of the experience—the emotional feelings and sensations in our bodies—is the painful part of the experience that we often try to avoid remembering and hold in our bodies.

While centering the awareness on inner feelings, we asked people to reflect backwards in time and find an earlier time in their lives when they felt the same way. Our experience in counseling was similar to what Janoe and Janoe found in their counseling in the 1970s with emotional feelings arising from present day issues and reported in *Dealing with Feelings Via Real Recollections*. They observed that emotionally charged issues triggered unresolved feelings from the past. By expressing the feelings around the unresolved issue and reflecting on these feelings, backwards in time, they found that people found the sources of their confusion and suffering in the present. These emotions were triggered in the present experience to signal to the person that they needed to reflect upon the past issues in their lives to free themselves from past-unresolved feelings. This perspective is also found in Jung's theory of complexes, presented in his *Collected Works Volume 8*, which views events as triggering the affects of early childhood events.

We found that it was through the process of reflection on inner somatic feelings, which were triggered in the present issue, that the source of the feelings causing the confusion and difficulties was identified. For the people we were counseling, the experiences in the present seemed to tie directly to childhood experiences through the awareness of their inner feelings. And these feelings, rather than the details of external events, seemed to be the accurate record of the impact of life experience.

It was our observation that it was not until these feelings were validated by another person as acceptable human feelings that people could begin to let go of the past and put their full awareness and energy into the present. We found that until the time people experienced empathy and validation for their feelings, they experienced themselves as being stuck in their earlier assessments of themselves with externalized thinking judgments as dominant. With the feelings and thinking still based on experiences from the past, the person did not fully experience the present moment.

Becoming Conscious of Inner Needs through the Somatic Reflection Process

We often found that if people reflected on an emotion in the present—like guilt or fear—and traced it back to an earlier time in their life, it was originally experienced with a profound presence of emptiness. For many people this emptiness was held deep within the body's memory. In working with people who had been abused in early childhood, Dr. Alice Miller writes in 1990 in *Banished Knowledge: Facing Childhood Injuries* that she found that people stored the memory of abuse in their body even if they were unconscious of it. In the present, the emptiness that our clients felt often seemed to be unconscious, similar to sensations and emotions that are cut off from awareness during trauma as observed in the work of psycho-physiological trauma theorist and practitioner Dr. Peter Levine. Often through reflection on somatic feelings, people became aware that the emptiness they were feeling related to the fact that their needs for acceptance and for freedom were not being met at that earlier time in their lives. That awareness had been stored in their bodies.

The awareness of their needs through reflection on feelings often helped people to see the reasons for their behaviors as children trying to fulfill their inner needs and overcome the emptiness of not having them met. They often found in reflection that the assessments they made as children about their behavior were ones that they were told by authorities in their lives. These new assessments of the reasons for their behavior were usually quite different from the ones they learned about themselves at the time of the early experiences.

Dr. Miller further speaks to this confusion of the child's assessment of early experience and the importance of a reassessment of childhood memories as one enters adulthood. She talks about the concept of "justified punishment".[26] She found that when adults reflected back with their minds only upon their childhood experiences of being abused, they felt guilt and blamed themselves for the abuse. Without the awareness of what they were feeling in their bodies and the impact of the trauma upon them, they attributed the reason for early childhood abuse as being necessary because they were bad and deserved the beating. She found that their abuser had afflicted this judgment upon them in early childhood. They had what she called "emotional blindness",[27] or a repression of their inner needs and emotional feelings in favor of an inaccurate judgment about themselves that they accepted from an external source, the abuser. However, when people engaged in a therapy that helped them get in touch with the emotional experience of these early abuses, they could reassess these judgments, identify the reason for the beating as the abuser's problem rather than their own as children, and accept their childhood feelings and needs.

Adlerian and narrative therapists Dr. Thomas Disque and Dr. James Bitter stressed the importance of connecting the awareness of the original emotional feeling experience stored in the body to the present thinking capacities, in order to reorganize the person's thinking about themselves. Through reflection back to earlier times in life, they found that it became clear to people that a confused way of thinking about himself or herself often originated with a direct external view or judgment of who they were from authorities in their lives. Dr. Richard Miller, a Non-duality Psychotherapist, posits a similar view. Non-duality is defined as the lack of separation in awareness of one's being. It is an awareness of being without splitting the awareness of the body and mind. Dr. Miller speaks of conflict and suffering originating from a misperception of separation when "we take in as babies"[29] a "central introject"[30] or core belief that we have been "born as a separate body/mind"[31]. He states that this belief is "fostered upon and into us by our parents, educators, and the world at large".[32]

Through becoming aware of the inner life through somatic reflection, we found that people learned to reevaluate their judgments about themselves that were based on inaccurate assessments in their past. This allowed them to feel acceptance of who they had been and who they were in the present. Through the Somatic Reflection Process, people gained new insights into how they could have served their own needs in a more effective manner. They began to understand how they came to be confused by an external view of themselves that did not accurately describe the meaning of their behavior. While people began to take full responsibility for their lives, they remained free of blaming themselves for the actions that they took or did not take.

With this feeling of acceptance gained through the Somatic Reflection Process, people felt free again to be themselves and trust in themselves to make decisions in their lives. It was at this point that we found people began to experience a union of their thinking and feeling functions and an integration of their psyche. We found that people were able to then make career and other personal decisions that proved to be healthy in their lives.

The Somatic Reflection Process assisted people in becoming aware of their inner instinctual needs and in viewing themselves from an inner reference that focused on what the organism was trying to accomplish for itself. When the behavior of a person was viewed from an inner reference of the organism trying to obtain a balance of the two instinctual needs of acceptance and control, a new awareness of the inner essence of the person was experienced. No longer were the body and the mind split between an external view in one's thinking, and an internal view in one's inner feeling experience. This new awareness often brought a healing, with a feeling of fullness and an acceptance of oneself that unblocked energy that had been trapped in the body. This release of energy brought a greater reliance on internal authority and a decreased need for external authority. It brought a growing awareness of a feeling of inner calm, a release of life energy, a heightened feeling of responsibility for one's own life, and caring for others.

"Therapists who are attuned with being are less likely to believe that anything is fundamentally wrong or missing in their clients . . .. Instead of being goal oriented, they tend to trust in the unfolding process of self-discovery."

(John J. Prendergast, 2003, p. 97)

CHAPTER SIX:

FACILITATING THE SOMATIC REFLECTION PROCESS

We are happy to share in this chapter a detailed protocol as a guide for facilitating the Somatic Reflection Process. This is only a guideline and should be followed with the awareness of one's gut, feeling-centered, intelligence. Therefore the process will vary from facilitator to facilitator and session to session. We first published the Protocol for the Somatic Reflection Process in Somatics Magazine in 2008 and the editor, Eleanor Criswell Hanna, has graciously given us permission to reproduce that material in this book.

THREE TYPES OF FACILITATION

There are three ways that the Somatic Reflection Process is facilitated. It is facilitated with another person acting as a facilitator, an imaginary facilitator, or an inner facilitator. The following is an explanation of these three types of facilitation.

The Somatic Reflection Process with a Facilitator

The Somatic Reflection Process initially begins with an external guide called a facilitator, who guides the experience. The facilitator both guides the patient through the process and offers acceptance for feelings as another member of the human family. According to Dr. Carl Rogers,[1] one of the main functions of the facilitator is to provide empathy. In this way, the facilitator offers a safe, facilitative container in which to foster the client's self-awareness. Dr. Rogers further describes the experience of empathy of the therapist as accurately perceiving the internal frame of reference or inner experience of the person while keeping an awareness of a separate identity. This is accomplished through listening without judgment and through clarifying restatements of what the person has said. Another method that may be used is the sharing of the facilitator's own experience of the emotional and somatic feelings and inner needs that the person is expressing. This sharing of feelings provides the reflector, the person who is reflecting on feelings, with the awareness of being internally and emotionally similar to another human being, the facilitator. This experience of empathetic mirroring provides a deep sense of belonging as Perera describes in *Decent to the Goddess* and we found in our counseling work to be the key to the person feeling truly accepted.

The facilitator guides the reflector through the process by asking a series of questions. These questions are presented later in this chapter as the Somatic Reflection Process Protocol. The questions are designed to assist the reflector in identifying an unresolved issue in the present life that has a strong emotional or somatic feeling attached to it. The reflector is guided to describe the feeling and the personal impact of the issue; and then to go back in time to earlier felt memories of the same feeling. This process is similar to

Dr. Eugene Gendlin's technique of guiding the person through *focusing*[2] as a method of centering on the felt sense in the body. The facilitator assists the reflector in staying aware of feelings in the body and in exploring the earliest memory of those feeling. Questions are asked by the facilitator to guide the reflector in looking at the inner needs at the time of the early memory and in identifying how those needs were met or not met. The reflector is encouraged to stay with the feelings in the body to make these assessments.

The questions in the protocol are designed to guide the reflector in examining how assessments were made of the reflector's behavior and what, if any, external authorities were involved in those assessments. The facilitator guides the process, but it is the reflector who makes meaning out of the experience. It has been said by Dr. Carl Jung that people rarely integrate what someone else tells them.[3] In depth process, interpretations will probably only be accepted if they come from the person's own awareness.

The Somatic Reflection Process is similar to a Non-Dual approach to therapy in that the foundation of both approaches rest upon the experience of the facilitator and reflector as present together without judgment. In both approaches, an inquiry guides the reflector from the "mind's interpretation back to direct, bodily felt experience".[4] Questions in both of these inquiries are designed to lead people to the "background awareness"[5] of their true self, the authentic being that is not a product of the mental constructs that people use to define themselves in terms of their relationship to the world.

In the final stages of the Somatic Reflection Process, the facilitator guides the reflector in bringing the awareness of the early somatic memory and the meaning of that experience to look at the present unresolved issue. The reflector can generally see that the conflict that has emerged in the present is an old one that relates to the same inner needs that were buried in the unconscious during early childhood. Often, the reflector feels more in the present moment and senses that a burden of misconceptions from the past has been lifted.

The Somatic Reflection Process with an Imaginary Facilitator

Once the Somatic Reflection Process has been experienced with a facilitator, the reflector can use an imaginary facilitator to ask questions about inner feelings. Holding the image of a facilitator, either the original facilitator or someone else, the reflector uses the same line of questioning and restating as was used by the original facilitator.

Facing the unconscious feels like a "dangerous enterprise"[6] when it is done alone. After 1978, we were not working together in the same vicinity and decided to continue using the Somatic Reflection Process with ourselves individually—each on our own. We found it helpful to imagine that we were talking to each other. We each became the imaginary facilitator for the other. We had the feeling as we individually imagined that we were talking to each other that we were not alone. This in itself had a calming, healing affect upon each of us. This process of reflection works similarly to active imagination and dialoguing with an inner figure. We have found that valuable intuitive insights emerge from the imaginary facilitator over which we do not have a sense of logical control. We are convinced that these insights have come from the unconscious.

The Somatic Reflection Process with an Inner Facilitator

There is a third way to experience the process in which the facilitator is completely internalized. The reflector has an inner conversation in the first person using the same line of questioning as with the original facilitator; but there is no personal image anchoring the facilitation. The conversation is with oneself. The person asks internally the same questions as in the Somatic Reflection Process protocol, and thus, acting as an inner facilitator, guides oneself through the process. For instance, one may ask, "How do I feel?" The person may then express inner feelings, in answer to this, by saying, "I feel empty and alone."

This conversation with oneself, using the inner facilitator to guide the process, is similar to what Dr. Fritz Perls calls in his Gestalt Therapy the self-regulatory nature of the person. With the use of "I" in the inner dialogue, he views the organism as achieving its own balance. External thought patterns are replaced by our own wisdom. For instance, when using the first person to talk about how one feels in the body, people find that they can understand what they need without *an external interference*[7], or another person to regulate their behavior.

After just one experience with an external guide or facilitator, people can, and usually do in our experience continue the Somatic Reflection Process by themselves either using an imaginary facilitator or their own inner facilitator. People would often say that after the initial experience with the Somatic Reflection Process, they surprisingly found themselves reflecting while doing a repetitive task like washing the dishes. This means that they continued the process unconsciously and were using the inner facilitator.

BEING ATTUNED AS A FACILITATOR: EMPTY MIND—FULL BELLY

In order to be attuned with the Somatic Reflection Process, the facilitator must learn to listen to one's own instinctual feelings in the body. Dr. John Prendergast posits a similar idea concerning therapists who perform Non-dual Psychotherapy. "Therapists will not be able to invite their clients to experience the truth of their being or the intimate touch of awakeness unless they have done so themselves".[8]

Psychotherapist Dr. Sheila Krystal suggests that Non-dual Psychotherapy is best performed by therapists who center on their "empty mind"[9] instead of their "inner commentary".[10] She finds it is essential that therapists listen with empty minds that have no agenda or judgment to change anything about the clients. By bringing to an empty mind the mental awareness of what the clients are describing, therapists can experience the issue without interjecting their own personal judgments that may change the meaning of the experience.

We propose a similar view in which the facilitator of the Somatic Reflection Process brings an empty mind and centers upon the gut feeling of fullness. The facilitator must enter into the process prior to meeting with the reflector, and come to a feeling of fullness in the gut area by previously working through unresolved issues using the Somatic Reflection Process. It is our experience that empty mind—full belly is the state of being that people experience when their instinctual needs are met for both acceptance and freedom. It is this state of being that we have found ourselves and others to experience when they are holding the tension of the opposites of acceptance and freedom. The facilitator must be able to clearly be in touch with inner somatic responses and be capable of staying aware of the authentic self within, experiencing a feeling of fullness in the belly. Non-dual psychotherapist Dr. Dorothy Hunt[11] is in agreement with this view and points out that therapist must feel the connection to the inner self or they can't hold the space for others to experience it. She further posits that if therapists are separated and split in their awareness of their minds and bodies, they cannot invite non-separation of the truth of their being for others.

At the same time that the facilitator holds an awareness of empty mind—full belly in the background of consciousness, there is awareness in the foreground of consciousness of the interaction with the reflector. By centering on gut feelings, the facilitator's own body can be used to gauge how a reflector may be feeling. We call this process *gauging*. We often found as facilitators that we got ideas or clues of what was important to ask the reflector as we centered on how we felt in our own bodies—particularly as we centered on the gut feelings of emptiness and fullness during gauging. Dr. Krystal supports this idea that therapists need to listen to their own "subtle psychic and intuitive cues"[12] that arise as they listen with empty minds to what is and is not being said by the clients.

While the facilitator is gauging the experience of the reflector, it is important not to identify with the experience. In the background of consciousness during gauging, the facilitator needs to keep an awareness of the centered state of one's own being with an empty mind and a full belly. Dr. Krystal discusses this same idea of therapists keeping the awareness of their inner sacred space and authentic self, or "resting in Presence"[13] while engaged in non-dual psychotherapy with clients. It is through holding this Presence that she posits that clients are "invited to a deeper level of reality beyond their belief systems, concepts, conditioning and tribal consciousness".[14] Similarly, we found that holding the empty mind—full belly state in the background of awareness, the facilitator may ultimately experience an empty mind—fully belly state in the gauging process concerning the feeling state of the reflector. The awareness of the sacred self that has been held in the background by the facilitator then moves to the foreground for both the facilitator and reflector.

Dr. Prendergast calls this process *sacred mirroring.*[15] It is a form of mirroring in which therapists stay in awareness of their own authentic self or "timeless dimension of being"[16] and share this with their clients. He views this experience of sacred mirroring as supporting the "phenomenon of a consciously shared field of awareness"[17] and as the state in which the deepest healing response occurs.

When we are aware through gauging that both our own self and the reflector are experiencing this state of empty mind—full belly, we have often experienced what the early twentieth century German theologian Rudolf Otto might have called a *numinous feeling*[17] or feeling of awe that is connected to the sacred. The numinous is the illuminated sense of the experience in an intense and uplifting way. Dr. Prendergast describes this same numinous quality with clients when he experiences sacred mirroring. As also defined in Non-dual Psychotherapy connecting sacred mirroring and the numinous feeling, we have often felt that this experience of the numinous during the Somatic Reflection Process is an indication that both the facilitator and reflector have experienced the healing process. Healing, the feeling of wholeness and the integration of the conscious and unconscious has come to both the facilitator and reflector through the connection to a greater whole or divine Presence that is experienced with the sharing of the awareness of the authentic self.

A PROTOCOL FOR
THE SOMATIC REFLECTION PROCESS

The following is a protocol of questions and responses for facilitating the Somatic Reflection Process. Although the questions are described in sequence, they are not necessarily sequential. It is important to view this protocol as a flexible guide and not feel limited to asking each question in the order it appears:

1. Can you identify the most unresolved issue in your life and center upon the feeling in your body that accompanies it? Where is this felt in your body?

2. Now notice what the issue is and the people involved in the issue that relate to your feelings. Are there any faces you see or sense? How do you feel in relation to these faces? Where is this feeling in your body?

3. How would you describe the feelings that you have concerning this issue? Please keep the details of the issue in your own mind as you describe the feelings.

4. Can you identify the feeling you described as being accompanied by a somatic feeling of emptiness or fullness in the hara (stomach) or solar plexus? If so, describe this feeling in your own words. (Occasionally, a reflector will start the process out with an awareness of a gut level feeling, rather than an emotional level feeling. In this case, it is only important to have them keep with the gut feeling they have described. Also if the reflector can not get in touch with their gut feelings at this step, have them go back and center on the

original emotional feeling they described in #3. In other words, assist the reflector in going to as deep a somatic feeling awareness as possible, but it is not necessary or advised to go any deeper than the reflector is willing to voluntarily go.)

5. Now, go back in time and remember when you felt this way before. You may wish to only go back only a few years ago, but this is up to you. Just see where it takes you. Now describe the feeling again and look again at the issue to see if it is the same issue as the one you started with. Describe it again. How does it feel in your body?

6. Now go back in time a little further and identify a previous time you felt this same feeling. Repeat directions for describing the feeling again as in #5, going back further and further slowly in time.

7. Continue to go back in time and repeat #6. Repeat again until you get to the earliest remembered experience of this same feeling and begin to have the reflector explore what the inner needs were at that time. Can you identify a need that you feel at this time in this experience for acceptance or a need for freedom and being in control of your own responses? Can you describe the feelings you had at this time? What do you feel in your hara and solar plexus? Do you have a feeling of emptiness or fullness that relates to these needs you described as being met or not met?

These last two questions of #7 are just for those who have not yet gotten to the awareness of their feelings in their hara and solar plexus. Often people do not get in touch with their gut feelings until the earliest remembered experience in childhood. Until that time they may only be able to center their awareness on emotional feelings like guilt or fear.

8. Are there external judgments placed upon you at this time around this experience from authorities and other significant people in your life—parents, teachers? What do you decide about yourself from these judgments? How does this feel in your body? Are you aware of your inner needs at this time concerning this issue? What do you decide about why you have these needs and feelings? From an awareness of your inner needs, do you have a different view of yourself now in reflection than you did then?

9. Now come back up in time and remember the original unresolved issue with which you began the process. Ask yourself if the awareness of seeing the past issue applies to this situation in any way. Can you see a similarity in terms of an inner awareness of needs? Can you see a relationship between this earliest feeling experience and the one in the present? Does it help to look at the present situation from the view of your inner needs from the past experience?

10. Can you describe how you feel now in your gut?

Identifying the Unresolved Issue and Feeling

It is often necessary for the facilitator to take some time with questions #1 through #4 in the protocol. If people do not have an unresolved issue that they become aware of quickly, the facilitator needs to define for them what is meant by the term an unresolved issue. The facilitator might say, "It is an issue that is getting in the way of living your life fully and happily, and if this one thing could be resolved, life would be much better, much easier." Or it might be easy enough to identify an unresolved issue as one that the person holds difficult or confusing or conflicting feelings around.

The facilitator asks the reflector to identify the unresolved issue and hold the awareness of the people and the situation in the reflector's own mind. The facilitator asks the reflector to center on just the feeling that arises as this issue or situation is thought about. If there has been no engagement in previous body/mind awareness depth-work and if there is no conscious emotional disturbance, the reflector may not have an accurate idea about what is meant by the word feelings. When many people are asked to describe the feelings that accompany an issue, they often will describe the story or details or a logical assessment of the value of the experience. It is important to spend some time assisting the reflector to find what the impact of the issue is and how it feels in the body. The facilitator needs to ask the reflector often, "Where do you feel this in your body?" The facilitator needs to have the reflector both say in words and point to the area of the body where the feeling occurs. Once the reflector understands that feelings are located in the body, thinking is experienced in the mind and the details of a story are what are happening outside of one's body, somatic reflection on body felt senses and feelings might begin.

We have found that there are some people who are immediately aware of their instinctual feelings of emptiness and fullness in the gut area, but the majority of people we have worked with are first aware of emotions that are located in the upper region of the gut and chest area. There is no need for the facilitator to worry about what feeling responses the reflector begins the process with. Often emotions like fear, anger, and guilt must be dealt with first, and they eventually lead the reflector to the awareness of a deeper level of instinctual feelings. As in question #4, it is helpful for the facilitator to often ask people what they feel in their gut area. But many times they will not be aware of those instinctual level responses and will wish to stay working on the awareness of emotional responses. It is always important to work with the feelings that the reflector is drawn to work with and to allow the reflector to feel in control of the reflection process, rather than to feel controlled by the facilitator.

It is also important to make a special note here that although a majority of people that we have worked with described the somatic feelings in the gut as "empty-full" feelings, other descriptive words may emerge from the reflector. I have had several people say that it feels like "yes" and "no" in the gut. And if we are working with a person whose native language is not English, we ask them to describe the feeling, if possible, in their native language and use those words. Even if they are adept at speaking English as a second language, this has been beneficial in helping persons to stay closer to feeling awareness in the body instead of translations of the head brain. We always respect the person's preferred way of naming feelings. It is, after all, the awareness of the feelings that is important, not the name.

Reflecting Backwards in Time with Feelings

Questions #5 through #7 in the protocol are designed to assist the facilitator in reflecting backwards in time with the reflector. After the reflector has located the feeling and personal impact of the issue, the facilitator asks the reflector to go back in time to an earlier period when the feeling was the same. The facilitator tells the reflector that it is necessary to only center on the feelings in the body and that the details of the experience they find in the past will probably be different from the original experience in the present.

The reflector is only looking for an earlier time when there was the same feeling, not necessarily the same details.

The facilitator tells the reflector that it is not necessary to go back in time very far. I have found that for many people, it is easier to get in touch with more recent feeling experiences first and then slowly make their way back to childhood feeling memories.

Once the reflector has found an example of a similar feeling experience that is in an earlier time in life, the facilitator has the reflector restate the feelings in that earlier experience. Again, it is important to have people keep the details of the story to themselves in their own minds and not speak the details. This helps the reflector get to the feelings by separating the impact of the experience from what was going on in the world around the person—the sensory data.

Sometimes, the restated feelings in this earlier childhood experience are perceived by the reflector as different from the original feelings expressed in the beginning of the session. In this case, it is generally because they have become aware of another feeling that is stronger than the first feeling stated in the beginning of the session. For example, a person may start out the session with the feeling of fear and anxiety in the present unresolved issue. The person may become aware in reflection on an earlier time when these feelings were felt that there is also a feeling of guilt accompanying the fear. The guilt may seem stronger than the fear. In that case, the facilitator goes with what seems to be the strongest emotion. The facilitator has the reflector restate the feeling and reflect further back in time to an earlier experience of that same feeling. In the example cited, the facilitator would ask the reflector to go back in time with the feeling of guilt, rather than the initial feeling of fear.

After the reflector has restated the emotional feeling that is being reflected upon, it is also important that the facilitator ask the reflector to be aware of any gut level feelings of emptiness or fullness. This is only to help bring the awareness of the reflector to those instinctual feelings. If the reflector is not able to become aware of these feelings, the facilitator continues working with the emotional feelings of which the reflector is aware. The facilitator continues to assist the reflector in going back in time with the same feeling until the reflector gets back in awareness to the earliest felt experience that can be remembered. Each time the reflector expresses finding another experience of that same feeling, the facilitator asks the reflector to restate the feeling.

Occasionally, people will go back immediately in this initial somatic reflection to the awareness of an early childhood experience. If they do, it is best for the facilitator to keep them reflecting in childhood, and it is certainly not necessary to jump back up to later life experiences to find missed examples of these same feelings. Eventually, it will be beneficial for the reflector to look at later life experiences with these same feelings and issues. That will help the reflector make sense of later experiences from an internal point of view. However initially, it is important to extensively explore early childhood where the feelings where first experienced.

Finding the Awareness of the Rejection of Inner Feelings and Needs

Questions in #8 in the protocol are designed to assist the facilitator in helping the reflector discover the inner needs experienced in childhood and the experience of rejecting the inner feelings concerning these needs. Once the reflector has a keen understanding of how to be aware of the felt experience, it can be helpful to begin to talk a little more about the details of the experience. The facilitator can judge whether the person can keep the thread of feeling awareness and still talk about the details.

We found that most people do this well once they are reflecting upon felt experiences that happened to them before age six—prior to going to first grade. Most of the details are simple and revolve around memories of the presence or absence of the main caregiver. Because the reflector has the mind of an adult, it is a common experience to evaluate the situation differently than as a child.

The facilitator is always listening and somatically gauging how the reflector is feeling. It may be the first time anyone has ever listened and understood how the reflector felt. Because the facilitator is somatically gauging, experiencing empathic listening and allowing themselves to have the feelings that they imagine the reflector to be having, the facilitator will seem very present to the reflector. And, in fact, the facilitator will be very present. The facilitator makes statements about how the experience feels and these statements are made as if the facilitator is speaking as the reflector. For example, if the facilitator understands through somatic gauging that the reflector is feeling alone and empty, the facilitator states, "It feels so alone and empty."

Of course, it is reasonable to assume that the facilitator will occasionally not gauge the reflectors feelings correctly as somatic gauging is a projection method, but the reflector is encouraged to make corrections and restate feelings as this occurs. At least, this has always been our experience. If the facilitator is aware that a feeling response cannot be clearly understood through gauging, the statement becomes a question, "How does it feel?" It is just as important for the facilitator to somatically understand how the client feels as the client. And without that empathetic understanding, we have found that little healing can take place for the client.

While reflecting on their feelings in childhood with the mind of an adult, people usually understand and identify their inner needs as children. They also can begin to see the decisions that they made as children to accept externalized thinking judgments (viewing themselves from the outside) that identified and then dismissed their own inner feelings and needs as being unimportant. It is therefore important that the facilitator often restate the needs of the reflector as they are expressed. It is helpful for the facilitator to ask the reflector to identify the needs and take notice of whether these needs were met or not. The facilitator asks the reflector what they decided about themselves when these needs were not met. Often the reflector will express a personal core belief about themselves that was formed in childhood around an event in which these needs were not met. It is important for the reflector to talk about this core belief and to identify the feelings that accompany it. It is also important to identify how the reflector originally came to decide this core belief. Was this a belief that the mind of a child decided about itself as it tried to figure out why it was not getting what it needed, or why it was behaving in a certain way to try to get what it needed?

We have often found that people can get in touch with their instinctual somatic feelings of emptiness at this early time of their lives even if they have not been able to do so previously. It is important that the reflector has a chance to feel into the depth of the empty feelings experienced at this early time. The facilitator assists the reflector in staying aware of this feeling in the body as long as needed for the reflector to feel validated that another human being understands that this is a perfectly human response and a perfectly human need. Allowing the awareness of this deep feeling of emptiness with the presence of another human being brings about a feeling of acceptance for the authentic Self or the core of our being.

Connecting the Feelings of the Past to the Present Life Issue

Questions in #9 and #10 in the protocol are designed to assist the facilitator in helping the reflector discover how the feeling awareness of the past felt experience relates to the feeling awareness of the present issue.

People can usually see for themselves the patterns of life experiences revolving around whether their inner needs and feelings were met and accepted. It is usually helpful for the facilitator to discuss the awareness of these needs and feelings in terms of acceptance and control/freedom of one's own responses. This concept of the felt experience of holding the tension of opposites around the need for acceptance and feeling in control of one's own responses provides a useful model to help people to understand themselves. If the facilitator has not talked about this model by now, it would be useful to do so at this closing experience of the process. It is important for the reflector not only to access inner instinctual feelings but also to have a way of thinking about these feelings that brings awareness and validation to what it means to experience the authentic Self. We might say that this helps link the head and gut brains in a cooperative association, and it is our experience that intuition and creativity flow at their peak when this link is finally made.

"The instinctual repertoire of the human organism includes a deep biological knowing which, given the opportunity to do so, can and will guide the process of healing trauma."

(P. A. Levine, 1997, p. 7)

CHAPTER SEVEN:

A RESEARCH EXPLORATION ON THE PERSONAL VALUE OF THE SOMATIC REFLECTION PROCESS

In 2005, an exploration was conducted of the Somatic Reflection Process using a depth inquiry with five research participants who volunteered from the graduate department of psychology at Sonoma State University (Love, 2005). We published a summary of that study in *Somatics Magazine* in 2008 and the following is a revision of that article.

Three of the research participants were females and two were males, with a variety of age levels represented. The purpose of this exploration was to discover if there are any significant themes and results that are valuable to the well being of people engaged in the process.

The research participants were asked to identify an unresolved issue in their lives, upon which the Somatic Reflection Process was focused, leading the reflector back into the awareness of childhood unresolved feelings. Two of the participants have given their permission to allow the transcripts of their actual Somatic Reflection Process work to be included as the last two sections of this chapter, as examples for study of the use of the SRP. It is suggested that the reader take the time to read these two reflections as they are real life feeling accounts that give the experience of the Somatic Reflection Process much better than hundreds of pages of discussing it from a more logical awareness. The names and some personal details have been changed for the anonymity of the research participants, but the feelings and general process is verbatim.

After following the Somatic Reflection Process Protocol, the facilitator then conducted a tape-recorded interview of the participants designed to explore the personal value of the process to the participants. All follow-up interviews in this study began with the following questions: How would you express the impact of this experience upon you? Did this process help you see anything new about yourself that you did not already know?

Three main themes emerged from the responses of the research participants to the follow-up interview questions. These were: increased somatic awareness; increased insights and new perspectives concerning inner needs and unresolved issues; and increased self-acceptance.

INCREASED SOMATIC AWARENESS

Several participants reported having an increase in somatic awareness. This included sub themes of feeling better in their bodies as a result of the reflection work and being more aware than before of what their bodily feelings were.

Feeling Better

One female participant, Cindy (all participants were given pseudo names to protect their privacy), reported that she "felt better" and had "slept better" the night following her participation with the Somatic Reflection Process than she had in a long time. She indicated that she experienced "a lessening of the original fear" in the unresolved issue due to the new understanding that it was an old issue and feeling. The following is an exert from the tape recorded interview:

> *The feeling—I didn't connect it to the longer view. And so that was the impact of this process; seeing that this wasn't a new feeling—that this was a very old feeling. The issue isn't as life or death [as I felt], knowing that it has happened again and again and again. So, there's a lot of lessening of the fear around it.*

Another participant, Steven expressed that he felt "lighter" and "really good" after the reflection process. He also indicated that the process "relieved tension." Similarly, Clea, a young female in her 20s, expressed a sense of "comfort" from the experience of the Somatic Reflection Process.

Increase of Awareness of Feelings in the Body

Another female participant, Sara, indicated that she experienced her feelings in her body while engaged in the Somatic Reflection Process. "It reached deep emotionally in my body." In an informal communication two weeks after the process, she volunteered that she continued the process automatically with an *inner facilitator.* She found further examples in early childhood of experiences of deep feelings, as well as somatic awareness of aloneness and emptiness concerning the issues of acceptance.

Bill, a male participant in his forties, indicated that the process had a "healing quality" and that he became aware of himself in his body on levels that he had not experienced using other "less body and feeling awareness processes" in the past.

> *It helped me understand things in degrees. Like seeing the degree and depth and amount of things [in myself]—it is one thing to say, oh my life has had such trauma; it is another to actually feel it in an embodied and conscious way so there is new— like fresh eyes experiencing. ...*

Clea indicated that the Somatic Reflection Process helped her "understand how to identify feelings and resistance to being aware of them."

Increased Self-Awareness

All five participants reported greater self-awareness. They reported increased insight into the issues they were dealing with, as well as increased awareness of their own inner needs.

INCREASED INSIGHTS

Participants said that the Somatic Reflection Process gave them a new way to view the problem or inner issue they were struggling with in the present.

New Perspective

Cindy reported that she felt the process was leading her to new ways of solving her problem with "a new perspective."

Sara commented, "It definitely gave me a new perspective that I think will help me toward resolving the issue. It helped me identify the dynamics and what my abilities are in solving the issue."

Steven expressed that the internal conflict he was having "got clearer" and that the Somatic Reflection Process gave him "a new direction." Steven further explained that it was helpful to see where the inner conflicts originated in childhood and how they had repeated throughout his life. "I never realized before where the conflict was coming from and how what I was feeling was really old." He expressed a deeper awareness of his psyche. "All of these voices are parts of me, and even if they are imposed on me and how I am supposed to be—at least now I know where they are coming from."

Bill indicated that the process was "very useful" in understanding the painful feelings he was having in the present. He expressed the insights he had as he reflected upon childhood from the view of an adult observer.

> *The best part was seeing it with the eyes of an adult rather than a child. I thought at one moment—God, people should do this regularly because I was visiting stuff that had frozen me. I had no idea as a child what or why these things happened to me, but now I'm an adult, and it's remarkable to sit with that contrast. It has a remarkable healing quality.*

Clea indicated that it was a helpful new perspective to identify a pattern of behavior that originated in early childhood experiences and has repeated in the unresolved issue in her present life.

> *It [The Somatic Reflection Process] did give me a new perspective about withholding communications. It's something that I have been realizing but I didn't realize what a pattern it was. I would pretend or deny [my feelings] and basically lie to myself and then to others. I was trying not to feel. So I couldn't tell others. [The Somatic Reflection Process] made me see the history of the pattern [of how I withdraw my*

feelings]. I see that I have done this pattern before and that is something that I hadn't clearly looked at. So to see the pattern is helpful.

Increased Awareness of Inner Needs

The five participants also expressed that the Somatic Reflection Process helped them in identifying inner needs and awareness.

Cindy reported that by participating in the Somatic Reflection Process she was able to become aware of her inner feelings. "It allowed me to feel how it had been so long since I had been truly authentic. "

Sara expressed, "I understand more where I am coming from. I see myself located in the issue now. Before, it was just happening to me, I now see myself internally."

Steven reported that he could see that often he did not experience a sense of acceptance from others for his feelings. He expressed this awareness when he said, "My whole life I have been expected to feel a certain way." He indicated that he was not able to feel the way people expected him to feel; he often thought he was judged for intentions and feelings that he did not have.

Bill indicated that he understood through the experience of Somatic Reflection Process that he had a greater need for freedom than he did for acceptance. "I think I've always gone for the freedom and ended up needing acceptance. An outsider would say I'm digging my heels in foolishly. Loss of freedom is the worse for me. I'll always show that in unconscious ways." He also found that attention to, and acceptance of, inner feelings from another human being are a basic need that he experienced during the Somatic Reflection Process. When speaking about the impact of the process he said, "This was so personal and I think this is what human beings basically need and deserve."

Clea indicated that she learned to accept her inner feeling responses as valid indications of needs:

> *I think that it emphasized to honor that I am sensitive. And I don't want to pretend and feel guilty and think that I am unfriendly or [have] a bad quality. I think this helped me know my boundaries and respect them. I use to think I had to change that, but maybe I don't. Acceptance is the biggest thing I feel coming out of this.*

INCREASED SELF-ACCEPTANCE

Three of the five participants reported increased feelings of self-acceptance.

Cindy communicated that the day following her participation in the Somatic Reflection Process, she awoke "feeling happy" about herself. She reported that she continued the process automatically with an *inner facilitator;* she had found further examples of how she dealt with her fears successfully.

Sara stated that the process helped her accept her needs in relationship with others. "I need to feel loved for who I am genuinely instead of what I can do for them."

> *Clea expressed gaining increased compassion for herself and acceptance of her feelings. She pointed out a benefit of her experience with the Somatic Reflection Process: "I think I'm getting on my own side and [being] supportive of myself." She indicated that the experience of the Somatic Reflection Process helped her "feel validated." Clea further expressed feelings of*

self-acceptance when she stated that, "It is comforting that my feelings were real and natural and not a product of being odd. I did feel odd— like an oddball. I feel more okay and accepting about being odd."

SOMATIC REFLECTION PROCESS OF RESEARCHER SUBJECT: CINDY

The following is an example of the use of the Somatic Reflection Process with a facilitator to deal with an issue in the present of an adult having severe anxiety in prospect of going for a job interview. The reflection reveals how religious judgments by family members devastated the patient as a little girl and how she carried this anxiety all her life. This person realized very young that these religious judgments about her were inaccurate and turned to nature and the out of doors for the acceptance she did not get from her family and religion. Still, the impact of the family religious judgments were devastating on her sense of self and has effected her all her life—both consciously and unconsciously.

Facilitator: Find in your own life the most unresolved issue in your life. All through this process, I don't really need details—the story—because we are trying to get down to the feelings and sometimes the stories make it difficult to get down there to the feelings. There will be times that we open the story up, particular when you are young and not in an adult-life situation. Sometimes before five or really young it can help to look at some of the details...But for the most part, we're not looking for details. So just pick the issue that first comes up to you when I say "what is the most unresolved issue in your life?" So just look at what comes up to you and say it to yourself, not out loud. Look to see if there are any faces that come up with the issue, with the feelings. You don't have to tell me that, just look at them in your own mind. And as you look at the issue in your mind, try to get a body feeling. Try to get a feeling somewhere in your body, how it feels—the impact of this issue on you. Does anything come up?

Cindy: Yes.

F. Can you state the issue from an inner meaning and feeling? Not from what someone might see but how you feel about it.

C. When you said that, I actually got a statement and the statement was "I don't belong here." The feeling is sort of frantic, not really frantic, but I don't know what to do, nervousness, in my stomach.

F. Would you say that this nervousness is anxiety—a little fear?

C. Yes, not a fear, an anxiety about what to do since this is true.

F. "I don't belong here and there is something that I need to do about it." This is in your thinking?

C. Yes, It's kind of like, I don't belong here but I'm here. So what I am I going to do?

F. And the feeling? It you say it is in your stomach and is an uneasiness?

C. It's a tightness.

F. A gut knot?

C. Yes. A knot. I'm anxious and when it's stirring my mind talks on and on about what am I going to do about it.

F. Frantic thinking?

C. Yes, like a panic.

F. So would you say that feeling is between your navel and solar plexus?

C. It's where my waistband is.

F. So right above your navel?

C. Yes. Right here (points).

F. Okay, so the feeling is uneasiness in that area—so lets take the feeling and go back in time, a fairly recent time when you felt it....

C. Yes, I have it already. I feel the same knot.

F. Okay, now center on that feeling and go back in time further, you don't need to tell me any details.

C. (Pause) Yes, I feel it at work, around a job.

F. And it feels the same?

C. Yes.

F. Okay, now go back with that feeling much further.

C. It's at another job. Just on the day that I get laid off. I don't know I'm going to get laid off but I feel this same feeling of being anxious. I think there is something that I need to do, I don't know what it is.

F. So that you won't get laid off?

C. Yes. To be allowed to stay there, I think.

F. So there is something that I need to do here so that I have a place here, but I don't know what?

C. Yes. And I can go back from there.

F. Okay. Go back with the feeling.

C. I'm there.

F. What is the feeling? It might help to see a face that is involved and get a feeling from it.

C. All the faces are staring... I have to walk through all these people who know I shouldn't be there.

F. And what is the feeling?

C. That same sick feeling in my stomach. I feel like I should have something to say if they stop me.

F. You might get judged?

C. They will know that I'm not supposed to be there— that I'm different.

F. Different from the others? You might get rejected?

C. Yes. These people are very rich.

F. So, let's go back with that same feeling.

C. Okay, I'm about 16...

F. What's the feeling?

C. Totally bad. I thought they were my friends. But sometimes this happens when there are three instead of two of us. I don't ever know how to fix that.

F. What is happening there?

C. I'm sitting in the car waiting for them. I know they will come eventually.

F. You are waiting in the car because it is cold or raining?

C. Yes, cold.

F. And you are sitting there looking at the house, hoping they will come out.

C. Yes. But, I know they will, they won't leave me out all night, they are just playing.

F. So the feeling is like being left out in the cold. You are on the outside.

C. Yes.

F. Do you feel that still down in your gut?

C. Yes,

F. So take that feeling, just the feeling and go back further in time to when you felt that way before.

C. Yes, in junior high.

F. Can you go back further with it?

C. In one particular class—the first day of kindergarten.

F. Why did you go to school?

C. I knew it was time and I went to learn to read.

F. You wanted to learn to read?

C. I didn't want to, it was time to.

F. Oh, you went to please mother?

C. Everybody went and it was time.

F. Mother said that everyone had to go?

C. Yes.

F. So how did you feel at kindergarten?

C. I was very frightened, there were a bunch of kids there.

F. Did you have that same gut feeling when you immediately walked in the door?

C. Yes. I didn't want my mother to go, but she did.

F. You mean that you didn't want her to leave you?

C. I didn't want to stay there alone. I wanted to all go back home and forget about it. (laughter)

F. And what did you feel when she left.

C. I was really afraid.

F. What were you afraid of?

C. I was afraid of all the children. I had never been with children.

F. You had never played with other children?

C. No, except at the doctor's office while we were waiting. And I always ran away because they were mean.

F. Do you remember ever playing with another child before school?

C. Once, a baby came up while I was at the doctor's office.

F. That was okay?

C. Yea.

F. Can you take that feeling of fear the first day of school and go further back in time before school?

C. Okay. Yes.

F. How old are you?

C. About three.

F. What is the feeling?

C. Oh, I'm afraid, really afraid.

F. What is the situation?

C. I'm in the backyard and I see some children across the street. And they tell me to come across the street but I know I'm not suppose to go there. But I go over there. And, almost immediately, I feel myself raised from the ground by the head. And my mother's got my ear and my hair and dragging me back in the house.

F. And she said?

C. "You've really done it now. And you're going to hell. And Jesus doesn't love you anymore. He did before but he doesn't anymore. You really did it!"

F. And how did that feel?

C. I felt horrible that I was going to hell.

F. Fear?

C. Yea, sad too, because I was fond of Jesus. I didn't want him to not like me or hate me.

F. You felt guilty?

C. I felt bad that that would be so and I was confused as to why.

F. It didn't really make sense to you?

C. Yea, it didn't.

F. Were you going to hell because you had defied your mother?

C. No, that was just one of those things that she said you are going to hell for—crossing the road. I don't know (laughter). But she had never said that before. I didn't know you could go to hell for crossing the road.

F. It was a quick experience with the children? You weren't there long?

C. Yea, I never saw them again.

F. That was a very earlier lesson in what happens when you follow your feelings? Yanked up by your hair. Where do you feel it?

C. I feel it right here (pointing to gut). It was so shocking!

F. Is that the feeling that you started with?

C. Yea! It is.

F. That's an intense lesson in your body. Isn't it?

C. Yeah!

F. You had this experience when you wanted to play with other children but weren't allowed to, does it feel like your needs are met as a child?

C. It seemed fine. I don't remember anything else.

F. Where did you like to be—inside or outside the house?

C. Outside, I loved the back yard. I felt I belonged there, in the presence of nature. I felt a belonging to earth.

F. In the presence of nature? You were free and that was okay. But what would happen when you stepped inside the house?

C. I was pretty free inside.

F. When you went in the house, did you keep the presence of nature?

C. It wasn't as obvious. There were things in there that I liked. I liked learning things with mother and the radio was always on.

F. Did you play in your room?

C. No, I followed her around. Everything she did, she taught me how to do. After I got older, I was doing a lot of it. Saturday's were a real pain. I liked it when I was little. It was fun and there were things I loved to do. And she gardened outside. I remember picking berries.

F. Was there anyone else around? A grandmother?

C. No.

F. Pretty much just mother. And father was off to work?

C. Sometimes an aunt would visit. Not a lot. And that was fine. There was no uneasiness for me—except religion. That was the only stumbling block.

F. Why was that?

C. Because if you don't clean your room, you're going to hell.

F. There was a lot of guilt put on you?

C. She... I learned to be careful. And the consequences of not being careful, like crossing the road, were enormous. Eternal damnation.

F. Before crossing the road and having that big experience, you are saying that you were pretty good at learning Mom's rules and staying within them? So you don't have too many problems but occasionally you get caught by surprise?

C. Yea. But it changed that day on the road, because that night in my bed, Jesus told me it wasn't true that it was a sin. (Cindy then describes an experience of hearing the voice of Jesus at three and feeling unconditional love from that divine presence.) From then on the bible study part didn't work and I didn't listen any more. I had it from a higher authority that it wasn't true.

F. How did you feel in relation to mother after that?

C. That she was wrong about all that and that she may be wrong about other things. And that was the last day that I could be a regular Christian. I sat in Sunday School but I could never listen to fundamentalism. The belonging thing—I think it was the belonging thing. I didn't belong to that anymore.

F. How did that feel?

C. I felt alone because I didn't know anyone else that felt that way. But I wasn't really alone because of the presence in nature.

F. You felt okay about yourself but you didn't feel you belonged?

C. Yea.

F. That was your choice, your new discovery about what you had been told?

C. Yea, I guess it was.

F. Going back to the first day in kindergarten, did that feel the same? Not belonging?

C. Yes, but I was also afraid.

F. How did you cope with that—did it get better as you met friends?

C. I was really shy. I bonded with the teacher. And, I had so much time on my hands, I would practice jacks—I would stay up all night practicing jacks or yoyo or whatever and I got really good at that. That drew some people to me at recess for the first time.

F. So you learned very early that performing could get you people in your life?

C. Oh, yea! I didn't think about that.

F. You learned quickly, how to do things and get along, you learned the rules, the ropes quickly.

C. Yea, I think so. I didn't really have a problem until I went to school. I can see now what it must have been like. I had never been around other children. I never thought about what that must have meant.

F. Can you take the feeling of not belonging that you felt as a child and see if it sheds any light on what you are experiencing now?

C. I don't know if I can work so well at night like the new job requires—I think I'm going to be tired and people will be mad at me and not really like me. I may not have the energy.

F. Going into a new job seems overwhelming? Do I really have the energy to get people to like me again? I'm anxious about it.

C. Yeah, that's the feeling, the knot in my stomach. I remember something (she laughs) about my last job.

(Cindy then recalls the story of how she nurtured people in her last job and was successful in making many friends. She seemed to find her natural talent for nurturing people and feel good about it as a skill that was something she always had and still had.)

F. What is the feeling about that memory?

C. Joy, relief of tension. I forgot that I did a good job, was creative, in my last job of getting people to like me, and I never really gave myself credit for it.

F. How is your stomach now?

C. Relaxed, really! I think I am way too hard on myself.

F. We all seem to drag around our judgments that we learned when we were young about ourselves.

C. I've looked at my childhood days before but I never got to the feelings in the same way. It feels good.

SOMATIC REFLECTION PROCESS OF RESEARCHER SUBJECT: SARA

The following is an example of the use of the Somatic Reflection Process with a facilitator to deal with an issue in the present of an adult experiencing a feeling of profound sadness. The reflection reveals how she discovers that she is not expressing her needs to others in fear that she will be rejected, based on experiences and feelings she is still carrying from childhood isolation in a family dealing with substance abuse by one of her parents.

Facilitator: Sara, you mentioned that you have an issue that you would like to explore, can you state that issue in your feelings, in other words, look at the issue and get in touch with your feelings about that issue and express those feelings?

Sara: (Shakes head)

F: Can you get in your mind the faces that are in the issue, but don't speak them just keep them in your mind? Then get a feeling you have about those faces and state the feeling—the impact upon you.

S. I'm sad and frustrated.

F: Can you describe in your body where you feel the sadness?

S: I feel the sadness in my heart, and I feel an emptiness in my belly.

F: Does it come from your belly and move up to your heart?

S: Yea. It's definitely grounded in my belly and my heart has a little piece of it [emptiness].

F: How does it feel in your heart?

S: It feels a little raw.

F: So, lets take those feelings back to a time when you felt them before. Center on just the feeling and go back in time when you felt it before.

S: Okay. Okay.

F: So how old are you?

S: 17.

F: Can you state the feeling again, Feel it and state it?

S: Yea. I'm frustrated and lonely—and really sad.

F: What's the sadness?

S: I think I'm sad because I really want to be with this person but there has always been something in the way.

F: You feel like it will never happen?

S: There are always complications and it's never at the depth I'd like it to be.

F: Can you go back with the sad feeling to an earlier time in which you felt that way?

S: Okay.

F: What is the feeling?

S: Sad. Empty.

F: Are there faces?

S: Yea.

F: More than one face?

S: Yea.

F: Is there emptiness?

S: Huh, yea. A total pit, it's very dark. (Stops to cry)

F: What are you sad about?

S: No matter how hard I try to be, I can never be what .... (pause), what is enough.

F: Not good enough?

S: No.

F: Do you decide what it is about you that's not good enough?

S: I can't figure it out? I try to think of everything.

F: You try everything and nothing works?

S: Yes.

F: How do you decide that? Is it because the person doesn't talk to you?

S: Because the person isn't loving toward me.

F: What does that mean?

S: There is a wall he puts up. I can't predict when that wall will be there.

F: Do you notice that he does this with other people or just with you?

S: Huh. Yes, there is one other.

F: That he does this with?

S: Yea. Actually, two more besides me.

F: Bring those faces in and see what you feel.

S: Angry and sad.

F: Are you still eight years old?

S: Yes.

F: What is the anger about?

S: I'm angry at this person, I don't know how to fix it.

F: Do you feel the emptiness then?

S: Not then, I just feel anger.

F: Why are you angry with this person?

S: My feelings of anger are for both my Dad and brother.

F: What were your feelings about your brother? Were they the same as you had in relation to your Dad?

S: There was a lot of difference between us. He seemed oblivious to everything going on.

F: How do you feel about him in that?

S: He just acts like everything is cool. I'm really pissed at him. He's just escaping.

F: What do you want him to see?

S: That our family is messed up.

F: How does that make you feel? Alone, for seeing this by yourself?

S: Yes. I take care of my Dad while my brother just spaces out.

F: And where is that felt in your body?

S: Here, all over really, in the solar plexus and angry here (points to chest).

F: Where is mother?

S: Huh.

F: Try to feel her presence.

S: I can't depend on her for any help. I don't know why I have to take care of him. I pretty much cut her out of my mind.

F: What is the most intense feeling at that time for you?

S: Sadness.

F: What do you do with this sadness?

S: I stuff in down in my belly. There's nothing I can do with it. Crying won't help.

F: Stuff it?

S: Yea, it's pretty strong. (facial expression shows sadness, grabs tissue, looks down at stomach)

F: Let's take that sadness and go back with it to a time you felt that earlier. Had you felt that sadness before eight years old? Can you find an earlier time you felt that way?

S: (long pause) It's hard to go back with it. I don't really remember before that.

F: Does that seem like the first time you felt that way?

S: I don't know. I keep getting pictures of my house that I grew up in.

F: Is that before eight?

S: Yea. As far back as a baby.

F: Where are you when you get this picture of you house?

S: Inside the living room.

F: When you center on sadness, it takes you to that image?

S: Yes.

F: Are you there alone?

S: Huh.

F: What are you doing?

S: It's the first time I remember feeling abandoned by my mom.

F: What's the feeling?

S: Terror! Utterly alone and empty. Terrified!

F: You are alone and abandoned?

S: Yea! It's interesting, I never saw before that I use to be very dependent on my Mom.

F: If you feel like it, you could talk about the circumstances back at that time of this event.

S: I was inside the house by myself and I had hurt myself in some way. I cried to my Mom. She eventually came running to my side.

F: How did it feel?

S: Totally empty. Laying on my back crying.

F: Do you get up?

S: No.

F: Had you felt that before, that feeling of abandonment and alone and empty?

S: It seemed like it. But I don't think so.

F: Can you go back further with the feeling?

S: Okay, I think I am alone in my bed. I feel the emptiness. I think I will have to take care of myself and be strong.

F: Why is that?

S: I just know it. I just know, I don't know, I know I have to be strong for everyone else. I have to take care of myself so they don't have to worry about it. It's my job in the family.

F: Can you come back up to the present situation with the feelings you had as a child and relate them to the present issue.

S: The feeling of unacceptable to my father, yea, it is the same, I feel unacknowledged and unappreciated. I feel so good inside myself with my own energy. Like I feel beautiful inside but no one gives a shit. People want to hurt it. Not love it. No one has ever really known me and loved me. No one has taken the time. No one who has loved me has really known me. It feels like love is never going to happen. I've pretty much given up that people will love me back. Whenever, I feel anything for another person, I'll just cut the feeling off. I don't trust it. I always did my own thing and that upset people. I was selfish according to others. (She describes experience of her dad being mad at her for not taking care of family when she was young))

F: There was a judgment from Dad that you didn't care about the rest of the family?

S: I'm selfish

F; So that is being unlovable, if you put your needs above theirs?

S: I usually put their needs above mine, but the minute I care for what I need and don't do things for them, when I'm not considering what they think, when I follow my thinking rather than their thinking, then they say I'm not considerate and I'm selfish.

F: When you do what you think is important, what happens.

S: They don't get there needs met. When I have needs.. It seems like the only way I can form a relationship with someone is to give to them. Because their needs must be satisfied and they only want to be with someone who will do that. I cut people out a lot because I get tired of it. I want to give equally. I can see that I learned that really young. F: Do you think you can use this understanding in the present?

S: I see it happening _ me doing it still.

F: Are you saying that you are seeing now a relationship between learning as a child to take care of other people's needs rather than your own needs and what you are feeling sad about—the emptiness you first described _ today?

S: Yes, I think I am still trying to, you know, satisfy other people. I don't even show people what I need—I don't even show me.

F: Maybe we could spend some time talking more about what you need.

CONCLUDING REMARKS

The Somatic Reflection Process warrants much more study as a somatic, depth psychology process that could be used to assist people in returning to an awareness of the authentic Self and finding the strength within toward healing the trauma of the body/mind split. This process seems particularly useful as a depth method because it engages both the body and mind, focusing on body awareness. It is also a process that once learned somatically, may be used as a daily practice by the individual for dealing with life traumas and unsettling experiences.

Both the clinical experiences and research we have done with this process supports the idea that it may be valuable in healing people experiencing trauma and stress caused by both emotional and physical conditions. The range of trauma that this process is successful in dealing with may well include the large number of returning veterans of the Iraqi and

Afghanistan Wars who are experiencing severe trauma and PTSD, as well as the uncomfortable feelings of accumulated trauma experienced by the common everyday hero living in our constantly-changing, stress-ridden, modern world.

The Somatic Reflection Process both encourages and gives support to understanding the authentic Self as we open the mysterious doors of our unconscious. Having a theoretical model and process of understanding our human inner needs and instinctual feelings makes it possible to integrate what we learn somatically about ourselves, thus supporting the communication and integration of the body/mind. As Gershon (1998) might suggest, it enhances the communication between the head brain and the gut brain and thus reduces stress and stimulates the intuition.

We have found that the Somatic Reflection Process is a technique for safely walking consciously into the awareness of one's unconscious somatic awareness. It's exploration as a tool is for anyone who is interested in recognizing and identifying the field of consciousness that is calling from deep within all of us, beaconing us to know ourselves as both individuals and as a human family, each with a human body with universal human needs and instincts that are at the core also caring for and connected to all of life.

There is nothing that can be changed more completely than human nature when the job is taken in hand early enough.
George Bernard Shaw (1856-1950) Irish writer.

CHAPTER EIGHT:

NATURE'S WAY

In this chapter, we attempt to expand the understanding of the principles of our nature's way underlying the Somatic Reflection Process and to also encompass feelings about socially related, institutional traumas to human needs. We will address the historical development of our use of external over-control of human beings in our modern world, showing through the ages how we got to where we are with our misconceptions of human nature, and the sense of false acceptance we have traded for true inner instinctive acceptance and well being as human beings and as a human family.

We would be remiss if we did not examine more thoroughly how we discovered through a step by step process, increment by increment, the integral calculus of our inner intelligence, which produced a piece of human understanding. We have presented the process of reflection as our fundamental tool used to produce the answers we have found within ourselves. Yet this tool, is now an external result of more than one inner principle, which nature has provided for use in the outside world. We will metaphorically examine some of these inner principles we can identify from experience, before we go on, as some of Nature's Ways.

There seems to be a natural principle in nature's achievements of adding-on to whatever has been achieved, whatever works. Nature doesn't scrap the progress it has made and start over, unless the results develop a fatal flaw. Examples of success are the Conservation Energy, Evolution and Gravity. Closely allied are the principles of electrical energy, magnetism, chemistry, physics, biology etc. a plethoras of forms of energy all existing together at the same time, 'waiting' to produce another species of energy when conditions are favorable. Nature seems to provide the unseen energy—with sub atomic particles—with the potential for visible new forms of energy, which can sustain the energy potential yet be used as long as the new forms are self-fullfilling with minimal or no loss of energy in the process. Thus it will support the new form—add on to its structure as long as that structure can maintain its self. Life is one of those spontaneous forms. Animal life is one of those mobile forms. Human life seems to be of that same ilk but is failing to utilize its given potential. It seems to be unable to control its cognitive skills from destroying its body. If the body isn't used as designed, in time it will be unable to sustain or reproduce its Self. This is a metaphor that explains stress and tightness in the gut.

The great mistake we have made with our intellect is to think we were created first, then everything else was created later to serve our needs. While we can be excused for not being able to see inside of ourselves to see the inner evidence of need in the past, we cannot be excused for not feeling the connection of the misery we have been causing to our-Selves.

We have been viewing our world backwards. The Garden of life came first and we came along later to enjoy the fruits and tend the Garden with the paradigms of caring, given to us as a result of the prevailing order. We were endowed with the wisdom of our species, which is far in excess of any other species, and we are provided with a brain to protect us, and everyone and anything else out there, from the chaos that still exists. Unless we can reverse our perspective now with a new image of our Humanity and operate from the center of inner intelligence—the wisdom of the ages—we will continue to let life be defined by external values, which have already marginalized human nature far too long.

The only way out of this pervasive human crisis is for all of us to focus our attention more on our inner feeling needs, give time to dwell (reflect) on any aspect of the past that will need the attention of our thinking intellect, decide what course of action needs to be taken, then turn over the action to the senses to lead the course of action in the outside world. This simple exercise of the intuition over time can provide the best decisions you can make by yourself. If this exercise doesn't work for you—doesn't satisfy your needs, doesn't produce a full feeling in your gut—then it is wise to share your dilemma with another person you trust.

It is best to use the Somatic Reflection Process for personal issues to adjust misunderstandings of the past and avoid the use of exclusive thinking intelligence. And it is best to use the intuitive processes for issues of movement into the future. The intuition requires the use of the thinking processes and the wisdom of the feeling intelligence together. These selective processes provide us with the best care we can find within ourselves from moment to moment. If we then follow the response of the gut empty/full signals, and maintain a reasonable balance of the two, life will get more satisfying, we will maintain the best health we can from within, and we will have plenty of energy for the care of others. A simple way of describing this exercise is:

"OPERATE YOUR INDIVIDUAL LIFE FROM THE INSIDE/OUT INSTEAD OF THE OUTSIDE/IN, AND TEACH OTHERS TO DO THE SAME!"

NEUROSCIENCE CHANGES OUR WAY OF VIEWING OURSELVES AND OUR RELATIONSHIP TO OTHERS

The paradigm of the individual's inner intuition, which seems to have been copied from our inner nature for cultural use, is perhaps due for more careful scrutiny. Something seems to go-wrong, when the use of human inner needs satisfaction—Acceptance and Control—is attempted in a group. Everyone seems to have their own idea of necessity, and after long wrangling and fighting, the only solution achieved is a compromise for everyone; no one is generally ever completely satisfied with the result. Is this an inevitable consequence? If it is, then the postulate of Acceptance and Control—the species basic needs requirements beyond food. water, and air—leaves many partly empty individual human lives, and the emptiness is reflected in the dynamics of the group. But how is this emptiness overcome in a group?

One obvious factor of group emptiness is that every individual in a collective is in the outside world of every other individual, therefore, each is perceived by the main brain through the senses. This is a tricky perception for we know that the main-brain is subject to errors of judgment of others, when based on observable behavior of others, and the accumulated experience of the perceiver's own past. And, we know that our observable individual, unique, external qualities also can separate us from each other. Each person has the inner needs prescribed by the species but the group as a unit often operates with the logical thinking process, with or without the conscious judgment of the somatic feeling process. Therefore, there is a reasonable chance in group activities, some social intercourse, will lack the presence of the inner somatic feelings, human nature's basic operating system, resulting in an inaccurate impression from experience and appearance. If the one observed speaks and incorporates his inner feelings, the observer's feelings can be triggered to respond to affect a more positive change in judgment of the observer. If there is no feeling spoken, there will be no softening of the original impression based on the impact of previous experience and appearance. The same dynamics applies with the involvement of the other senses—that of taste, touch, and smell.

Put in historical perspective, social intercourse has been operating in many western cultures with the assumption that the instincts of human beings should be suppressed as children age toward puberty in order to become acceptable social animals as adults. This doctrinal dogma seems to have intensified as people have congregated in cities, where time spent in freedom is severely diminished and where encounters with differences in looks, speaking and behaviors in people are common experience.

Acceptance is more difficult in the urban setting because of the differences that often fail to meet our expectations. This causes emphasis in our encounters with each other, to be placed on sensed differences rather than on our common, instinctive humanity. The differences among us tend to cause grouping around the principle of like social characteristics and ideologies. We form exclusive communities, clubs, churches, schools, and political-affiliations, even cemeteries, with the expectation of greater satisfaction from affiliations with other like-minded individuals. These folkways and mores are, we believe, examples of groupings relative to the instinctive need for more Acceptance—an indication of a feeling of individual emptiness.

There are other potentially more sinister reasons for grouping that result from the perceived need for instinctive Control. But in this case, rather than applied to self-control, the action becomes the control of others. We use the adjective, sinister, because this misuse of the control of individuals and groups by external influences have little or no concern for individual instinctive needs satisfaction, but for power, prestige, or economic benefit for themselves, or small exclusive groups or again distrust of human nature. These ideologies are also possible indicators of empty lives that cause further emptiness of the society at large, emptiness due to the loss of individual Freedom, the human foundation of Acceptance and Self-control, triggered in the present by unresolved guilt of the past.

We don't think it's necessary to detail the history of mismanagement of instinctive human needs in order to relate to the cost of emptiness in human lives. Recorded history of 'civilization' is crowded with examples of lives lost, energy expended, and resources wasted for individuals to gain back freedom from oppressors. This 'rebellion' seems to occur when life is becoming less important than Freedom to be one's Self, and be Accepted for needing to be able to control one's own time and space. There is a limit to human-adaptability that requires distraction of the organism away from basic human needs satisfaction, and this limit seems to be gauged at the stabilizing somatic feeling level. The influence of the enteric nervous system seems to be quite adaptable, but sometimes life can be too empty for the basic operating system to support life.

There is one beautiful example of an analogy that mimics the use of the functional Thinking/Feeling relationship we have been talking about in a group setting, which has a good chance of achieving satisfaction of the instinctive human need for Control and Acceptance. Remember, there are two brains, one brain focused on the outside world and the other brain focused on inner body operations, and each brain is functionally independent and has its own special purpose. When each brain carries out its function, referenced to the organismic needs, the organism operates as a single unit and the unit grows and matures successfully according to nature's plan. On the other hand, if the thoughts of the main brain are distracted, by its sensory information, away from needs satisfaction of the unit, the second brain responds with the intensity of feelings appropriate to the degree of distraction. If this distraction from the unit's needs continues, dysfunction sets in and some sort of crisis will occur. We are including the respective nervous systems of each brain, and the constant dialog between the two systems, in this analogue.

We are all familiar with couples living together, either in our own relationship or as an observing child. There is usually one partner whose primary job, in relation to the needs of the family, is to focus his or her thoughts and energy primarily on the world outside, and express those thoughts to the other partner. There is usually another partner whose primary job is to concern his or her self with the inner needs of the family and express those feelings to the other partner about what's happening in the home. When each one carries out her or his assignment, referenced to each other's needs, the family operates as a unit, and the family grows and matures successfully according to nature's plan. This use of a paradigm of natural distinct roles in the outside world, a human-made design, is almost an exact copy of the instinctive nature of each individual in the relationship.

Even the feedback loop of constant dialogue between the two separate, independently functional systems is necessary for the stability of a family. This feedback between members of a group seems to be necessary in any relationship where a group is working toward a common goal, if the goal is to be successfully achieved. The inner feedback, the internal dialogue between the main and second-brain, provides the process by which human instinct directs itself toward the future, and the instinct with the recorded past experience of the organism's intuition, informs the upper brain of the logical possibilities for common needs satisfaction in the future.

In a group, the intuitive process is working within each individual, but the individual intuitive-results depend on the experience factor, the nurture of each individual. The variation in the experience factor (nurture) seems to be responsible for the separation quality in the intuitive exchange, resulting in disagreement, but the constant dialogue has the quality of healing disagreement if both thinking and inner-feelings are present, regardless of the different nurturing experience of the individuals.

A person learns and understands from sharing instinctive feelings with another person who accepts and communicates the same feelings that he or she is the same instinctively as the other fellow human being. But ultimately for optimal needs satisfaction and good health, the person needs at least two other people with which to share innermost instinctive feelings. With one other sharer, the person feels much better about him or herself—feels less alone and less odd, but the person may still think that he or she and the one shared with are just two odd people in the world. However with a third person coming in on the sharing, we have found that the person feels that he or she is a part of a group, a family, a human family. And it is then that we feel most perfectly human.

We could equate this to something every pilot knows. If you are flying an airplane and you need to know where you are, you need two signals coming into your instrument monitor. If you only get one radar signal, you will not have a fix on where you are and you best hope that your visibility is clear enough to eyeball your locality, by way of what you see on the ground. But with two strong signals coming in, the pilot knows exactly where he or she is, and the crossing center vertex is established. The human psyche is similar, in that with two strong signals from two other people communicated to us indicating that we are the same in instinctive feelings, we have a complete sense of who we are inside and no longer feel lost, alone and empty. It is for this reason that we have always felt it important to reflect with people in groups of at least three.

It may be important to begin reflecting with a person with just the two of you, but as soon as it is comfortable to do so, it is very wise to open the experience to three or more. This is quite a different group experience that we are suggesting, we would like to add, than the group dynamics where people are interacting directly with each other on feelings about each other. Our approach, even with issues between two people, has always been to have each person take the responsibility for his and her own feelings and go back into time with the reflection centering on what feelings are being triggered in from past experience with an emphases on clearing the past to be more in the now. Generally, this yields enough understanding that people are able to better communicate their needs and relate to each other in the now; and with this approach there is little need for a group encounter with negative feeling exchanges. Once people hear each other's feeling stories, they most generally feel empathy naturally and instinctively for each other and work to find ways to better communicate what they need from each other so that the group as a whole may benefit.

INTIMACY AND INSTINCTUAL GUT RESPONSES

Intimacy is suggested between individuals in a group when the inner qualities of the basic operating system of somatic feeling is employed with the thinking process of the main brain. But the image produced by the word "intimacy" has become confused with sexual activity for many individuals. It seems to be forgotten that intimacy is an essential quality of the nurturing process in childhood between the young child and other members of a family.

In a caring family, intimacy becomes part of neurological growth, which prepares a child for adulthood, and seems to be associated with the process of acceptance and control, the basic operating system. Intimacy may be seen as an objective of the process of finding the likeness of one's self in others. Intimacy may even be seen as learning about one's self from others. In other words, it seems to invite others into a closer relationship to experience a genuine feeling of self-exposure that would lead to genuine acceptance. This experience of intimacy is like having a very close friend, whom we can trust with our thoughts and feelings about anything, without judgment or offence, the kind of relationship we would never risk loosing. Then why do people tend to associate intimacy with sexual activity, regardless of whether sharing feeling awareness has occurred or not?

Again we go back to the state of basic instinctual needs satisfaction of individuals. When we examine the sensory intake of the main-brain and the negative attitudes of many toward the human instincts, along with the absence of feeling awareness of the human basic operating system, we likely find empty lives. It is no wonder that people in emptiness confuse closeness in spatial relationships with closeness in time and meaning that is felt and shared.

Dr. Gershon[1] suggests that the discovery of the gut's center of intelligence, *the Second Brain*, provides a threshold for a Renaissance in the field of medical practice, since study of the animal digestive system has been avoided and taken for granted in the past. A similar change in the dynamics of intra-personal relationships may be called for in order to adjust our lives toward what they were designed to be. That design seems to have been ignored causing nature's plan to sail off-course at the peril of the species. The adjustment to somatic feeling awareness requires a blank, open mind about the image of reality with which we are faced.

THE LANGUAGE OF THE GUT:
ME, MYSELF, AND I

There are multitudes of examples of the use of the thinking-feeling paradigm in the growth of the art of mobility. This intuitive art must have been used early in human existence when it was first discovered that walking and running upright had advantages over lumbering along on all fours. When erect, man could see objects further away and could carry objects in the hands. People could hide or circumvent danger to avoid conflict, or they could use the same skills to gather or capture food. These new experiences produced neurological growth in the central nervous system of the upper brain and the enteric nervous system of the gut. The history of that growth seems to have been stored in each nervous system in the language appropriate to each system. The upper brain recorded information in the language of the sensory data it received from experience—that's Me. The gut record was of the same experiences, but recorded in the simple language of Empty/Full, representing needs of the organism—that's being My Self. And when there was action and we move as a unit, it is recorded as I, I said it, I did it, or sometimes, I didn't do it.

These three identifiers, Me, Myself, and I, have been used through out memory, especially in those experiences of extreme Emptying or Filling qualities. It seems that we have always had a notion that Me and Myself were often in dialogue, either agreeing or disagreeing, trying to work in concert, so that "I" could act in a manner that would change "my" gut gage to stop moving toward empty and move toward full. We are reminded of the little fellow we call "conscience" sitting on the shoulder of a person who is arguing for the opposite sides of a decision—Me and Myself were trying to resolve an issue to act or think as one, I will or

I will not! This little picture represents a subconscious awareness of the enteric nervous system in action, and this is the signal Dr. Michael Gershon identifies as "Butterflies in the Stomach". It seems obvious that we—me, myself and I— knew the information had been stored to be used in a moment of need, to clear up a problem the three of us were facing. We could use past experience as a reference to move into the future and to implement an idea that could make life more meaningful. We think this process is called Intuition.

MOBILITY AND THE GUT

As humans found the need to roam further and further distances, the idea of a beast-of-burden came into their minds to simplify mobility, and to carry them, and their possessions, wherever they needed to move. As the human world expanded, so did their use of their thinking/feeling skills, and, with increased use of intuition, the thinking/feeling paradigm became a major functional characteristic of the species, requiring a larger more neurologically complicated head and body than was needed initially. According to Dr. Lise Eliot the motion function is one of the earliest developments of the newborn human organism.

It has been suggested through neurobiological research that the adaptability of the human organism was the result of the two separate neurological systems, the main upper brain and the gut brain, in constant dialog. Even though physically and functionally separated, these centers of intelligence are interconnected in such a manner to allow the organism to move as a single unit. It was also found from clinical studies, that both intelligence centers contributed to a learning process, which allowed the organism to store the data from an experience and be prepared to meet future happenings that together they could imagine might occur. In other words the organism was able to learn from the combined experience of the two brains, and use that learning for future possibilities. It was concluded from this information that this phenomenon was the source of the human ability to reflect on the somatic feeling data of the past and adjust the true meaning of past experience—the impact of past experience on the organism. This would allow the somatic feeling experience of the gut, along with the details of the sensory system's experience to engage in intuitive learning processes. This phenomenon seems to be characteristic of life of the mobile organisms that have been equipped with variations in design to adjust to varying physical environments down through the ages. The success of this security system has been adequately demonstrated, in part, by the longevity of the species and the growth in complexity of the system. The growth also permitted this thinking/feeling combination to be used in a wide variety of nonhuman applications.

Another aspect of the presence and the functional relationship of the two brains is the thinking/feeling paradigm, which has provided for the organism to develop more abstract possibilities, as man's brains have grown to handle more complex information. Originally, it appears that the combination of the two intelligence centers was the source of a security signal for mobility—whether to stay and fight for its freedom to be in a space, or to run for its life when the odds for survival were questionable. As man's world of experience has expanded, so too has the size and capabilities of the two brains, to accommodate his ever changing ideas of mobility.

Where mobility is perceived to be a need, adaptability is required. Adaptability provides learning. Learning results in Evolution. Evolution opens the centers of intelligence to new possibilities, and so on, and so on....

ADAPTABILITY AND THE GUT

It doesn't seem possible that the process of adapting could occur with only one center of intelligence, for the reason that the process of adaptability requires a dialogue between the center of reference and the center of prospect. Without the use of the two centers working together, no effective evaluation could be made. Without the perception of the upper brain, no idea of a prudent movement could exist; and without the supporting energy of the gut brain, mobility would not be possible. The only place where mobility can exist for man, without either or both of these two centers of intelligence, is in the environment of the mother's womb where DNA furnishes the intelligence and the mother's body provides the source of energy and support for mobility—at least initially. It is in the mother where this paradigm of two reliable centers of intelligence seems to be introduced and becomes an instinctual guide to human development.

We will try to demonstrate this adaptability principle using the paradigm of the two brains in a very common human development of the 20th Century, the Horseless Carriage—the Automobile. The only way a reliable direction for mobility could be possible for the carriage, without the horse, was to use the human brain to survey the surrounding landscape sitting in the carriage seat to guide the carriage and the horse. The intuitive possibilities of a horseless carriage removed the horse, with the horse's intelligence, from the front of the carriage. The engine must be mounted on the rear so the driver of the carriage could see where the carriage was heading. Without the intelligence of the horse to respond with his learning, both voice (GEE—HAU) and lines to pull (Right—Left) connected to the bit in his mouth, and voice commands (Get-e-up or Whoa-a) to command him to (Start or Stop), the intelligence of the driver and the design of the carriage would have to be adapted to take the place of the intelligence of the horse.

The engines, available at that time, were being used to propel boats and ships, and to provide energy for industrial plants, so applying that engine to the horseless carriage was a matter of developing the means of mounting and connecting. The matters of starting, stopping, and turning, the general problems of coordinating the intelligence of the driver and the intelligence built into the more complicated carriage, is an evolutionary process in itself. As we know, the evolution of the horseless carriage didn't stop there.

To quickly move the idea of the horseless carriage into the modern automobile is to pass over years of struggle with model after model, most of which are extinct, using the intelligence of past experience with the thinking/feeling of the human organism intuiting, in ever so small steps, over a period of more than a hundred years. Compare that process of developing the present model of the human being. It is likely that it took millions of years, increment by increment, to arrive at a model that could adapt to the changes and challenges of life. If we don't take care of our present human model, by using the brains with which we were born to support life, we may become part of the "scrap heap", that didn't use the brains they were born with and became extinct.

EVOLUTION AND THE GUT

The evolutionary process from the horse drawn carriage to the horseless carriage, a simple idea in the minds of late 19th century humans, is one of the myriad of evolutionary processes that not only relate to the mobility issue of man, but also reflects the instinctual involvement of two centers of intelligence, in dialogue, which provide a variety of intuitive possibilities for the future. Some of these possibilities may evolve into problems of mental health if we don't put some special effort to nourish human awareness of the original purpose of the somatic feelings. This will be true if the excitement of the upper brain continues to marginalize either of the basic human needs of control or acceptance.

For the person driving the horseless carriage, it was the intelligence of the upper human brain that was doing the thinking about where the carriage was going. If they were walking, the engine attached to the carriage body acted as an energy substitute for the gut energy available. These two functional centers of intelligence, mechanically connected for mobility to move as a single unit, raised the importance of the upper brain, with its nervous system, and diminished the importance of the gut, with its nervous system, so it seems. The inner feelings of the passenger, whose upper brain was less affected by the experience, was probably experiencing less loss of the inner feeling awareness of acceptance, but was experiencing an inner feeling awareness of diminished control.

The paradigm of nature seems to be the need for a balance between control and acceptance. Both driver and passenger would have experienced a better control-acceptance balance by walking. The beginning of the loss of awareness of the gut signals, and the overwhelming focus on the sensory data, seems to occur when we design substitutes for the gut responses that tend to smother the sensitivity of our instinctual feelings of our enteric nervous system. We tend to loose control of our security, or even worse, we set up the situation where the two brains are no longer able to establish adequate dialogue, or simply can't agree for healthy decision-making. This is an unfortunate scenario resulting in mental and physical illness, or even, over long periods of time, extinction of the species.

Remember that it is the ancient brain, with the enteric nervous system in the gut, guided by the DNA in every cell of the body,[2] that is the first system to be completed, tested and functioning after conception. It is the upper brain, with its central nervous system, that was left to develop itself, after birth.[3] The development of the upper brain turns out to be a function of the quality of care that the organism receives during the first few years of exposure. Combine the chance inherent in the DNA received at conception and the chance inherent in the quality of the care after a child is borne, it's a wonder that there are any 'standardized' qualities of human behavior. If it weren't for the process of "survival of the fittest", which works in the human realm as evolution— nature's experimental process, we would not have a dependable mobile species. If we, out of arrogance, ignorance or neglect, loose that dependable quality present in the definition of the species, it is entirely possible that we can look forward to evolution towards 'disasters in the making'.

INTUITION AND THE GUT

As we maintained in the evolution of the automobile, the ideas for these man-made devices, and in every case of invention of a system by man, there is an uncanny resemblance to the structure of the human intelligence systems and the evolution that follows the initial design, even in the detailed 'blueprint'. *We don't invent, we simply intuit the ideas from within ourselves.* Anyone can do it, if given the preparation. But unless we develop a more conscious awareness of nature's contribution to human survival— mobility, adaptability, intuition, and evolution of the species, we will slowly continue to move toward physical and mental illness. With conscious attention to the inner needs—our organic needs other than food, water, and air—as we continue to evolve and develop the things of commerce, comfort and convenience, we can better understand our present problems and intuit directions of health and satisfaction in life, and continue to be, *one of nature's successful species.*

When the intuition is used to satisfy a human need, energy is provided to fulfill the possibility of the full feeling in the gut, and the organism benefits. When the intuition is used to promote a head trip—something we desire in our thinking but don't need—the fantasy can soon disappear and be replaced with an empty gut feeling. We can seek after the un-necessary more and more as we loose contact with our gut feeling in favor of our sensory attractions of the outside world. Our view is that this action is producing an empty and sick society .

THE MATURING OF SCIENCE USHERS IN A NEW IMAGE OF HUMAN NATURE

Reflect back two or three thousand years ago and try to imagine curious minds, trying to describe the process of life and its beginnings. They would have drawn their conclusions from their life experiences, from their external observations of other's behavior, and their interpretation of what their senses recorded. As for what was going on inside the organism, the only source of answers to that physiological mystery had to be conceived and accepted from their own inner feeling experiences. The 'understanding' of their own inner nature would have had to be related to the necessity of the inner needs satisfaction of the species, which was experienced but yet unclear to them at that time—the acceptance of each other and the control of their daily lives. Since the lack of needs satisfaction of life over time was unbearable, the only source they could identify to mediate their intolerable existence on earth would logically be vague and otherworldly, the same mystical power in their minds that had created the world around them. As the centuries passed, faith in these otherworldly images became fixed; otherworldly power became their hope of salvation; prayer became communion with the mystical power, earthly practice became their collective faith; and nature's periodic relief became their miracles. Over time, these practices became accepted faith that human necessities would be furnished ultimately in another world after death. Life on earth must have been very difficult everywhere, for this pattern of inner need satisfaction from a mystical heavenly source became a universal phenomenon in the east, and middle east-in Persian, Greek, and Hebrew cultures.

Some time in the first five centuries A.D., as the Christian movement strengthened and spread, the Roman Empire conceived the idea that it could use these images of expressed need satisfaction to bolster the empire's control of its people. By establishing a center of conditional acceptance, the empire could control the masses and support their thinking towards otherworldly salvation, since pressures against the Christians to conform was not working. If the empire was able to modify the existing images of earthly freedom, with a promise of a better life after death for those who met their conditions, the empire could flourish. This center became the Roman Catholic Church, and was so successful with its doctrines and dogmas, that even though the empire was later destroyed, the Catholic Church lived on to perpetuate the faith in much of Europe, and later in America. Much of the power was gained by force in Europe and Great Britton, but was later lost in Britton and diminished in Europe due to the Protestant Reformation. Threats to the faith didn't destroy the need for a better life for the masses. Misery of disease, wars, natural catastrophe, fraud, oppression, and political corruption, still remained to support the perceived need for mediation, and allowed the institution of a church to spread westward, and take on a wide variety of denominational forms in North America, all derived from the same images of the faith promulgated by the Roman Church, yet adapted to the needs of attendant, diverse, and widespread congregations.[4]

We have tried to present a cursory bit of western historical perspective to put into context the scientific discoveries of the 20th Century, trying to avoid an arbitrary view with an unfair judgment of who possesses the truth. Science has matured to avoid an arbitrary view with an unfair judgment of who possesses the truth. Science has matured with its increased depth of understanding of the inner workings of the human body mainly due to the availability of materials, equipment, and knowledge. The details of tissues lying within the body could never have been examined if it hadn't been for modern technical developments-the Electron Micron Microscope, the DNA/RNA revelation, the x-ray, the MRI scanner, the EKGs, the Computer, advancements in Biology, Chemistry, Medicine, Physics, Engineering, Psychology, and the pervasive value of the Semiconductor. Perhaps all of the professions have allowed the inner human organism to reveal itself to curious human minds. Now medicine can describe some critical significant results of modern scientific research to offer more reasonable and more understandable images of the past mysteries—the same unknowns that seemed to have disturbed our forefathers.

The same dilemmas, but with more serious consequences, are facing us humans today. There are many more of us and many more attempts to control our thinking. There seems to be a need for us to seriously look back at our behavioral patterns and the images of our inner selves to improve our intra-personal and inter-personal relationships. We need to take a new look at what factors are responsible for our external behavior that seems to be getting us into greater trouble. Science is in the process of giving us some preventive and curative answers to health and environmental problems, which call for preventative and curative rethinking of the inner intelligence of the human species, and a rekindling of the conscious awareness of our own inner nature.

"Much of the inner, deep nature is therefore unconscious . . . . It persists underground, unconscious, even though denied and repressed."

(Abraham Maslow, 1968, p. 192)

CHAPTER NINE:

A NEW PSYCHOLOGY OF GUT INSTINCT

While we have demonstrated in both our personal counseling work and our research over the past four decades that the gut region of the body—the hara to the solar plexus area—is the source of the feeling aspect of all emotions, modern psychological thought does not yet give the gut this honor. There are those in the psychological field that now say feeling is in the gut and talk about gut feelings as a connection to the intuition, and that is certainly a start. But that is where it normally ends and we are left wondering how, why, where, when and what the gut is speaking about to you when we have a "gut feeling". Few talk about the voice of the gut. Is it really just talking about digestion of food? We have so many questions once we accept that the gut feeling in the stomach is worth investigating on a psychological level. Is it possible that the gut is trying to tell you what your psychological needs are as a human being?

Although there is a growing interest by self-help book writers and some therapists who have joined the life-coach movement—like Dr. Martha Beck (2011), monthly columnist for Oprah Magazine—who are pointing to the importance of following the awareness of gut instincts, there essentially is little real formal psychological theory of the gut at this time in modern accepted psychological academia and thought. Even those studying and talking about the link of intuition and the gut have been dancing around the psychological exploration of the instinctual nature of the intelligence of the gut response. Yet for some time, psychological theories in understanding the importance of the gut are briefly discussed in the literature of somatic practitioners like psychotherapist Dr. Eugene Gendlin, who talks in his book *Focusing* about the physical experience of the *felt sense* or internal sensations that include the gut feeling; psycho-physiological trauma expert Dr. Peter Levine and his work with the *frozen* energy in the nervous system resulting from early trauma experiences; along with other trauma experts like the late Dr. Maryanne Eckberg, who worked a number of years in El Salvador with the Commission on Human rights; and Dr. Bessek van der Kolk, who has been active as a clinician, researcher and teacher in the area of posttraumatic stress and related phenomena since the 1970s and works with sensation and the person's connection to the reptilian brain to learn to be fully engaged in the present rather than being haunted by the past.

While these therapies mentioned are reported to be quite successful, the voice of the gut is not specifically studied and thus these theories leave us with some questions about the intelligence of our self-regulatory system and instinctual needs. We learn through these somatic treatment approaches what the ingredients are that make up the self-regulatory system of the body, but we do not learn the source of the instinctual needs that the body protects. Through looking at the gut as the gauge for the instinctual needs and responses, we can begin to understand not just how we operate optimally in general, but who we are coded to be in our

DNA/RNA and where the source function for this coding is found.

THE VOICE OF THE GUT

In the four decades that we have worked with hundreds of people to understand the gut and its relationship to instinctual need, we have found some amazing, but we think really simple, truths about the gut responses, the gut voice, and about the nature of human beings and our instinctual needs. The gut response is simple, but it also can be complicated to understand within ourselves and by the time we get to be adults, we can barely recognize our gut responses. To understand them, we have to use what we can feel of them and reflect backwards in time centering on their feeling and recover our awareness of these responses. The external world, including any Freudian based psychology, will tell us to not waste our time doing so and that these feelings are unreliable, unimportant and if followed will lead us down a disastrous road. We understand that many people are frightened to make this internal exploration, so we only put this work out for people who feel called to do so. We have, however, never found anyone that was sorry for having explored his or her gut feelings. We do advise that before making your mind up about what you really think about your gut responses that you actually explore your feeling gut center carefully with the Somatic Reflection Process. It does take some work and without a true effort we can be lead astray by our thinking process and find more inaccurate evidence to blame our problems on our gut feelings. So this is no quick fix, but every minute we work at this will bring us closer to valuable self-awareness that will enhance our life quality.

In essence, if we were going to boil this down for someone who wanted a quick idea of what the new Gut

Psychology is, we would say that the gut is the instinctual response center and we feel either empty or full or somewhere in the middle (imagine a gas gauge) in our gut at all times. We feel full when our instinctual needs are met and empty when they are not. We are talking not just about food intake (although the feeling of emptiness and fullness in relation to food intake and psychological instinctual needs are interestingly similar and we do get them confused and thus may over eat to try to fill the emptiness we feel psychologically). We are talking about psychological instinctual needs—psychological not in the use of logic but in our needs as human beings. We have two instinctual needs that the gut gauges—the need to feel accepted and the need to be in control of our own responses to life. These two needs must be constantly in balance. Too much of one without the other leaves us empty. When we have both of these, we feel very full and thus energized; and when we have neither, we feel empty and often experience some symptoms of stress in the body like feeling lethargic, anxious, overwhelmed, disconnected and alone. This gut response does not depend on the thinking brain as the gut is an independent brain of its own (see Dr. Michael Gershon's research), but of course it can be greatly affected by the thinking brain, and vice-versa. We work both consciously and unconsciously to keep these two instinctual needs in balance at all times. Our understanding is simple and if we start using this as a premise for our thinking about our experiences with our feelings in everyday life, it begins to make a lot of things clear to us about our needs and motives and our human nature.

At best, we need to have a balanced and conscious dialog between our gut responses and head response so we can use our thinking brain to make the appropriate responses in the external world and try to fill these two important instinctual needs in appropriate and successful ways.

However, when we are unconscious of our gut responses, our thinking brain will often use a system of thought it has picked up (perhaps from an authority like a parent, teacher or even a religion) and applies it as a judgment about the feeling in our gut. This is what happens when we have an emotion like guilt or depression. We feel empty because our needs are not met and our thinking brain attaches a thought to the emptiness and lack of our fulfillment like "It is all my fault for being too stupid or too small or too incompetent, etc." or "I am not capable of doing anything to make this work or be better", thus we have guilt and or depression feelings. These emotional feelings are not pure feelings of emptiness or fullness anymore, as they now have the thinking component mixed in them. And these thinking-feelings or emotions are mostly felt in other parts of our bodies above our hara, between our head brain and gut brain. If you look into your emotional feelings, you can always find a thinking element to them. And if you trace the feeling aspect only, it goes directly and purely to the gut. For as we have said, the gut is the source of all feeling.

Generally, the only way we can unravel this tightly woven thread of inaccurate thinking judgment and resulting emotional stress, is to reflect back to the source of when the thinking head first applied this very same judgment and find the actual source or as close to it as possible. And the key to finding this first experience is through reflection on the gut feeling of emptiness and fullness, not through thinking back on the details of our lives. Once we find this original experience in which we started the "tape" that plays over and over in our heads that we are all at fault, powerless, too needy, unlovable, etc., then we can lift the sentence we have placed on ourselves and our feelings and begin to see ourselves clearer and make healthy decisions—begin to use our thinking head to follow our instinctual needs and fulfill our true human nature.

Of course, we realize that this is frightening for people because people have long ago been convinced that our human nature is selfishly uncaring and they, therefore, think that is why we need laws and religion to keep us in control (not that we are against laws to help us have a guide). Freud founded Psychoanalytical Psychology with statements of this lack of dependability of human nature and it is difficult to pry the human race away from this dark and inaccurate judgment of whom we think we are deep inside. As we reflect on somatic gut feelings and listen to the gut voice, we see that it is the very judgment against the consciousness of our human nature or our gut instinctual responses that is ultimately responsible for the evils that it preaches against. So while it may seem frightening at first to reflect on our gut responses, people like the caring person they find themselves to have always been when they reach the consciousness of the gut response. And becoming aware of one's true inner nature, instinctive gut feelings, is not generally thought by those who experience it to be in conflict with the essence of one's spiritual knowledge, but more of a Gnostic direct experience of the Sacred experienced in the gut or all of nature that is greater than us and is connected to us through the gut instincts. Some call this experiencing Presence.

Reflection on the gut voice helps us to be more mindful of our caring nature and thus be more caring for others. And with the new awareness of our gut responses and needs that we acquire through reflection on our instinctual gut responses, we are able to live a more caring and healthy life with the thinking head finally conscious and listening more clearly to the responses of our most reliable and authentic self—our gut instinctual feelings in our body. What is called in yoga chakras systems as the Nabhi chakra located at the hara or gut center will fill and overflow with energy to the Anahatha or heart center and it will open with compassion loving others and improving the feeling of well being and the strength of the physical immune system.

GUT EXPERIENCE

We now have developed a new image of human nature, with which we can offer a clearer understanding of human intellectual potential based on the modern medical research in neuroscience and cell biology. Dr. Michael Gershon has opened a new door for how we think of ourselves, validating a new Psychology of the Gut, with his research and breakthrough discovery of the gut brain. His research focuses on the enteric nervous system (ENS), and the intrinsic innervations of the bowel as a part of the peripheral nervous system that is capable of mediating reflex behavior when input is absence from the head brain or spinal cord. This medical discovery leads us to the understanding that human beings have at least two distinct brains or sources of intelligence. Mankind has possessed this gut brain intelligence for ages, but has been encouraged not to trust it, not to use it because it was associated with human instincts. By inference and even more direct, this intelligence was considered evil by nearly every branch of society. When children reach an age of social understanding, or even earlier they are taught that the root of evil rested with the instincts, even though some serious thought would realize, it was the same instinct, which had created human nature. By suppressing this essential intelligence, it was easy for societies to prove its evil theory, since when suppressed, we now know somatic feelings can make themselves known to social norms in highly disruptive ways. Without the guidance of the natural instincts, which are designed to be used in the human make-up—the DNA/RNA, the human animal's intelligence has been compromised in ways that produce behavior patterns similar to some of the lower animal species.

The importance of the suppression of this vital function has been taught, and that since the human being is something special in the animal kingdom, it achieves this standing by associating itself with an other-worldly center of intelligence for rules of appropriate thinking and for rules of appropriate behavior. Under this regimen, somatic inner feelings are in conflict with external thinking, and even though we humans are designed as something very special, it is not because we are using external patterns of thought, it is because we have the language skills that allow us to communicate with each other and experience somatic feelings of intimacy through dialogue, from which we learn who we are and how to relate to each other.

The new science challenges us to take a new look at individual and social human behavior, and to realize how attitudes about these instinctual qualities are affected. If we humans are to remain and prosper as healthy animals, we must understand what medical research is uncovering. From our experience with human behavior, in which we worked at the post high school levels of education in the 1970s, we have accepted the challenge to incorporate new medical science into a new Gut Psychology with a new image of human nature and project the affects that a new image of human nature would have on existing cultures.

Now validated by medical science in the studies of Dr. Michael Gershon, human nature has provided the individual with at least two centers of intelligence—two brains: One, the ancient animal brain, with its own nervous system with its domain in the gut and its own independent intelligence to produce the energy of life for the entire organism. And two, the sensory brain, that is the upper brain and the surveyor of the external world, looking for necessary actions for the human organism to survive and develop the sensory intelligence needed to cope with outside environments. The two brains must then learn, over time from experience, to coordinate the two separate intelligence functions to produce the energy of life while sustaining the human species in this outside world.

This image is a simplistic view of what we are and we have presented a functional image to remind ourselves of the potential each of us possess, to help us reflect on what can happen when we use these vital tools (thinking and feeling) to support life, or what happens when we ignore, forget, or fail to develop either center of intelligence, since we need them both to make healthy decisions. When we discuss the principles of human gut experience we must remember that in general, we humans are very much alike, but in the details of experience, each of us is unique and must develop our own personal methodology of solving problems, however minor such an adjustment in methodology might be. Each of us must learn to take care of our selves, to know and respect our strengths and weaknesses. We are conceived by accident by parents who likely met by accident, and who furnished the specific genes we have—without any knowledge of what they were contributing—by accident.

There is one grand plan of development, with precise timing and precise detail of the finished product, during the managing of the beginning of animal life, supporting the human organism as it develops toward birth, and will furnish energy to the entire system throughout its life span. This nervous system in each of us humans, or its equivalent in other animals, seems to have been perfected in such a manner that its intelligent function can be adapted to the needs of all animal species. The principal of its operation, furnished by a gene pool, seems to have the basic purpose of sustaining any form of life in an infinite variety of ways. Its intelligent adaptability creates life from the initial cell division for almost an infinite number of animal species. Then remains as a stabilizing influence during the species' life span, and seems to be the last aspect of life to die and degenerate after it has served its purpose.

We offer what may seem like an 'intuitive extreme' to make the point, that order and purpose seem to be a birth object, which creates this order out of the chaos of the universe and seems to furnish a *raison d'etre* for life. This source of intelligence, which seems to exists universally throughout the world in all forms of life, including we humans, seems to be successfully used to support its life form, seems to be utilized successfully by all forms of animal life except the human species. This error seems to be related to the power of the upper sensory brain's ability to take and store information, and its obsession with the nonessential aspects of the outside world of the senses (CNS), drawing attention away from the stabilizing influence and wisdom of the enteric nervous system (ENS) in the gut, or, we humans have yet to learn its value and how to use it. Perhaps there are still other possible reasons why we have failed to integrate this vital system into our vision of ourselves. It may be possible that we have never been free enough from external controls to develop the individual use of this system, or have used a faulty image to understand our selves. After all, individuality has not been supported even in our education system until recently, and not with support from some of our powerful institutions. We will likely learn in time that individuality must be turned on early so we are experienced enough with ourselves that we are able to guide our own learning in such a manner as to fit our own individual inner and cultural needs to keep our minds and bodies healthy (referring to the instincts of Control and Acceptance).

Problem Solving and Gut Instincts

Problem solving seems to be an art form, which requires elements of all time frames, the past, the present, and the future. Each frame of reference has its spatial images of the outside world of experience, set in time. And, each of the inner feelings, which we inevitably experience, represents the impact of that experience on our inner well being set in time, and the nature of art with its use of thinking, feeling, and reflection over time represents a human paradigm of nature's problem-solving.

The time frame of the past comes to present awareness only when in reflection we recognize it, however, it seems to influence at least unconsciously every action we take. While we do not necessarily focus on the past, the autonomic nervous system can furnish experiential information when it is needed and available. It is in this frame of reference which we have spent our forty years of work. If there is no clear enteric-system evidence in the present, then we must work our way back (reflecting with feeling) to the past relevant data in the past frame of reference, to the natural impact on the gut before a satisfactory solution to problems can finally be found. This Somatic Reflective Process (SRP) can provide us with the soundest course of action based on our understanding of the meaning of our past actions. The reports we receive from our upper brain, however, contain elements of outside world judgments and alone bring a minimal, if any, degree of satisfaction to solution of our inner needs. Only if we have been sensitized to be aware of our instincts earlier in life, can the instincts seem to motivate action of necessity to the organism. Thinking motivates action referenced to judgments of the impact on our minds of outside environments. Thus the action we take in decision-making depends on the guidance we are using, thinking from the CNS and feeling from the ENS—from a combination of both centers of intelligence on the same issue.

Elements of the present raise questions of degree of necessity of our inner needs as opposed to the pressure of sensory wants. The present is a time of action when we face issues which need to be addressed, a time when guilt—unresolved issues from the past meets the fears of the future—a time when we need all the intelligence we can muster. Unfortunately, this is not a prime time to call for the wisdom of feeling intelligence unless, of course, we have already learned how to temper the power of the senses, wanting some thing so much that the feeling-signal of simple need has little chance to compete with the stimulation of the senses. The present is a time when an awareness of inner necessity can easily be ignored or missing, a time when an over supply of sensory data will compound and not help us in our problem solving.

How important is this issue of an existing balance of need and want to present decision-making? The answer to that question is probably related to how much experience we have gained in the past with the degree of balance of our inner needs we have been able to sustain, how much past experience we have had, and how supportive of the organism the data has been. We define inner health as the balance of control of our time and space and our feeling of acceptance by those close to us. The presence of a close friend dispenses with a lot of want and shrinks many disturbances to a size that allows many problems to disappear entirely.

Elements of the future present us with the consequences of our actions. How will our actions affect us latter on, and those in our environments? Will we be taking too much control and risk acceptance, or will we be looking for too much acceptance to risk control? This is a process for the intuition, which requires all the intelligence available if the final action actually supports a genuine inner need—does the resolution of the issue fill us or empty us—the gut feeling response. Going into the future we need to be honest with ourselves.

If we focus on our upper brain alone, we will provide logically biased answers to problem solving, which, if action is taken with this evidence alone, will tend to leave the issue unresolved, with a major portion of external judgments and a disruptive gut response. Where as, if the reflection process includes awareness of the gut reaction—tightness of stomach muscles, sour stomach, tension, emptiness, etc, or a relaxed condition in the gut and a sense of fullness, and this data is incorporated in the considerations of necessity, the resolution of the problem can be made with confidence—whatever it is—that the action taken will be in the organism's best interest, even when the resolution of problems are contrary to thinking. As we learn to take the time to reflect on what both centers report, in all problem solving—the thinking intelligence of the upper brain and the feeling intelligence of the gut brain—we can achieve a peace-of-mind, less stress in the body, a more positive self-image, improved health, and lower doctor bills. It is yours for the little time it takes to develop the healthy habit of including the gut response to problem solving—the effort can become the healthy assurance that both centers of intelligence are being used in facing problems of your life, and regardless of the decision it is in the best interest of the organism.

There are at least two possible avenues for us as a culture to take, in support of human intelligence in society. We can develop the awareness of the two centers of intelligence in the education of children, so that the decision-making-experience represent what children learn through early experimentation, and avoid the early judgments of good and bad behavior, with less repair work to be done later to the self-esteem. Or we can continue to resort to corrective therapies when help is required, which is now the scheme only in theory, since it is not very effective without a more accurate human image. Corrective therapies tend to miss students who have the greatest need for attention, those who have dropped out of school or are dismissed from school for unacceptable behavior. By including both schemes, students in early grades will have been coached to manage their own social behavior among themselves, leaving many fewer students who will need and should receive in-depth corrective attention. We view early childhood Somatic Education as the most important application of Gut Psychology.

When we reflect on this human equation of self-control and self-acceptance, we see both the complexity and the simplicity of the problems, which lie ahead. We predict, however, along with the predictions of the founder of client-centered psychotherapy Dr Carl Rogers, that with the emphasis on innate intelligence in the education of the newborn, preschoolers, elementary, and beyond, we will have far less concerns with individual and collective human behavior problems later in life. If we take both the long term and the short-term approaches, most children will have developed a more positive self-image and better health, having learned self-control and self-acceptance through years of practice. Adults will learn to join in as the years of experience show results in children's behavior. We will find more student energy, more relaxed students, a cheaper more efficient, and a more effective education environment. This issue of the early learning of individual control and acceptance as an experiential subject represents the Renaissance of Education and Psychology, which Dr. Gershon predicted in 1998 for Medicine.

Renaissance: Freedom and Recognition of Instinctual Feeling Responses

We would like to use this historical metaphor, Renaissance, as an inner instinctual feeling awareness of human nature, which is sending a desperate message to its cognitive awareness. To paraphrase the message, "...you are deviating too far from your design objectives, your external and inner necessities. You are on a path of self destruction unless you can break the bonds of serfdom and gain the respect you deserve as human beings—now is the time to act to save yourself or die trying." Such a message as this emerges as an intuitive result of the disturbances of the periods of the Renaissance and the Enlightenment, which hints at the human nature involved but focuses most of the attention on what took place in external environments. This emphasis on the external world is the result of reflecting on the happenings of the past with the single brain image. On the other hand, using the two-brain image, we can interpret the total decision-making process as an inner phenomenon as well. This double brain process does not change the facts of history but it includes the reason for action (the logic) and the vital need for the risk (the feeling with the energy to accomplish change). What happens in the outside world are the results of human energy supporting individual and collective intuitive need, not just the social cause.

The entire process of human inspired events seems to take place and have a lasting value when there is something seeming to benefit the inner needs of the organism. When there is support from both 'houses' then there is furnished energy of motion, confidence of purpose in the intended result, and movement towards the objectives.

We can intuit the gradual emergence of the power of change of inner human need, control and acceptance, overpowering the external controls of feudal control. The two-brain image established by human nature has, up until now, lay partially hidden from its own understanding, subject to interpretation by external imaginations and external judgments. In the past, the external awareness of the possessor and observer alike accepted the presence of something internal existed but it didn't fit the ideas of external control. There existed something internal to all human beings that could be externally disruptive yet supportive, good yet evil, indifferent yet loving, dependable yet unreliable, certain yet unsure. It seems clear that this mystery became the prudence of the action of Charlemagne to incorporate the early Christian movement into the Roman Empire and form the Roman Catholic Church (RCC). The sequence of events that followed were understood and projected primarily as progress of intelligent adaptation to the environments, providing major contributions in wide ranging endeavors to existing cultures in Western Europe (printing, literature, art, science, philosophy, religion, etc.).

Consider the following quote about the meaning of the Renaissance from the *Encyclopedia Britannica*, Vol. 19, pp 222-223, 1958:

> Important as the Revival of Learning undoubtedly was, there are essential factors in the complex called the Renaissance with which it can only but remotely be connected. When we analyze the whole group of phenomena, which have to be considered, we perceive that some of the most essential have nothing or little to do with the recovery of the classics. These are, briefly speaking, the decay of those great fabrics, church and empire, which ruled the middle ages both as ideas and as realities; the development of nationalities and language; the enfeeblement of the feudal system...the Renaissance was rather the last stage of the middle ages emerging from ecclesiastical and feudal despotism, developing what was original in mediaeval ideas by the light of classic arts and letters, holding in itself the promise of the modern world. It was, therefore, a period and a process of transition, fusion, preparation, and a tentative endeavor. And just at this point the real importance of the Revival of Learning may be indicated. That discovery of the

classic past restored the confidence in their own faculties to men striving after spiritual freedom; revealed the continuity of history and the identity of human nature in spite of adverse creeds and different customs; held up for emulation master-works of literature, philosophy and art; provoked inquiry; encouraged criticism; shattered the narrow mental barriers imposed by mediaeval orthodoxy.

Humanism, a word, which form assumed by human self-esteem at that epoch—the ideal of life and civilization evolved will often recur in the ensuing paragraphs, denotes a specific bias, which the forces liberated in the Renaissance took from contact with the ancient world—the particular by the modern nations. It indicates the endeavor of man to reconstitute himself as a free being, not as a thrall of theological despotism, and the peculiar assistance he derived in the effort from Greek and Roman literature, the 'litterai humaniores', letters leaning rather to the side of man than divinity.

We have injected this bit of history of human struggle to make several important points. First and primary: Change seems to be supported and directed out of human necessity to be free—not be controlled by outside forces of any kind at any stage of development, which distract it from its instincts. Temporary excursions seem to be tolerated but never forgotten and constantly tested—just like an animal in a cage. Human nature has provided the intelligence to expend energy in a direction that will set us free—however long it takes, and whatever action is necessary. Second: The human's self-image seems to gain stature from asserting itself in support of the instincts of its species, and is not defined individually by casual judgments from those who are looking for something in return or for self-aggrandizement.

This combination of inner qualities seems to set the stage for the ability of each one of us to provide ethical behavior for positive social intercourse without control by any outside force. The pattern of possible inner self-control of our individual behavior, and the knowledge that the species is, or can be universally endowed with these qualities, opens a door to assurance and trust that if we spend the time long enough to understand each other well enough, we will provide support for each other within the means available. Even though it may be prudent for incremental change rather than total change at once, towards human inner need and freeing human energy, the essential ingredient of life itself is achieved when energy flows freely back and forth between each other.

"We cannot teach people anything, we can only help them discover it within themselves".

(by Galileo Galilee)

CHAPTER TEN:

THE NEW IMAGE OF HUMAN NATURE IN EDUCATION

To attempt to deal with education as a process of human need and health for the individual is to reverse our focus of attention from the plethora of external environments, to the inner world of human necessity and need, to the subject that is being revealed to us daily by scientific discovery. We are being alerted and warned by science that the direction that we are presently taking in the education process, and other elements of the culture, is not satisfying individual human nature. So far, we have ignored the warning signs, because such a change of human image from external control, to self-control and self-acceptance, requires a new image of human nature, which we previously defined to meet the requirements of a healthy mind and body, but does not fit into the present cultural plan for education.

The education plan that we have always used is our version of the British plan, which was designed to educate the public to provide labor for the industrial market place. This plan has provided an occasional mind full of curiosity and discovery, but for the general public school graduate, there is often little satisfaction in the occupational choices that the individual is forced to make. This occasional curious mind is most often not a product of the public education, per se, but the luck of family circumstances, or other personal circumstances, which elsewhere provided the environment for learning personal control and acceptance—the ingredients for a positive self image and the intuitive process of discovery.

Instead, throughout our culture we see examples of the distortion of the human need for personal control and personal acceptance. This distortion of necessity of human instincts, for the continued inner guidance of the unique individual life, results in external control and some form of exclusive acceptance of others. This distortion has caused the suppression of human instincts simply because, without the continued training of awareness of the early satisfaction of the inner needs, we have failed to provide the continued support for such human characteristics as positive self concept, ethical social behavior, and inexhaustible curiosity present at birth. All human strengths seem to have come from early practice and later experience with trial and learn in supportive environments.

THE LEARNING PROCESS

To approach the idea of the process of learning, we need to bring into the discussion the dual functions of *control and acceptance* and add still another set of dual qualities of awareness, the concepts of *prospect and retrospect*—future and past time, with the present now time squeezed in between. So, to review the variables with which we are now working we have the basic instinctual human needs, of *freedom/acceptance*; the inner feeling of *empty/full*—the gut gauge with its feeling record of *human needs satisfaction*, the data from *five senses* focused on the outside environment, the humans in it; the *Intuition,* and the collaborative results of past experience of the two intelligence centers working in concert. We also need to remember that the gut intelligence center can operate independent of the upper intelligence center at will.

There is at least one more point to remind us of what to expect in the use of our intuition in the learning process in our early life. Experience, in prospect, often has a large portion of feeling and a small portion of thinking, especially in our early years, when we may not have a wealth of thinking experience with which to work. In retrospect we find some authorities in our lives will have a logical, highly critical judgment of our action, leaving us with no possible explanation of why we took the action. This kind of experience puts the damper on freedom to take overt control of the individual life, and can cause irreparable damage to the self-image over time if continued, as well as the learning process in general.

Entering a new experience is most often perceived as an attractive prospect to our 'needs' satisfaction. Whether it is an inner human need or something that just attracts our senses, we can rationalize our attraction to it, that we will be more satisfied with having the experience or object than without it; the intuitive leap forward into the future in prospect, based on data or information we previously acquired from past experience. In our early youth, there is not much stored with which to intuit, not much with which to guide. Therefore, trial and learn is our key to our experience. Therefore acceptance by those in the environment is essential. Not much but guilt results from the advice of observers. This principle applies to any type of action we might take in the open or in private, verbal or physical.

Once acquired or experienced, the object takes on new meaning. Often our experience falls short of our expectations, and we wish we had given more consideration to having the experience before we acted. Sometimes we can correct the action and we forget it, with only a minor empty feeling in the gut. Other times we are stuck with unexpected, undesirable results, and the gut feeling we experience is sickening. Some intuitive leaps are with us for the rest of our lives. Why do we make these 'mistakes' if we possess all the intelligence we claim to have?

Remember, the enteric nervous system, connected to the ancient brain, is the only center of intelligence available to us at birth[1], with only the potential for the main brain and the central nervous system to develop from experimentation with its potential. What else but 'trial' and 'error' is available for learning? The design objectives are built into the cells, but there is no cognitive awareness of what path to take toward those objectives, except the time based incremental results of experimentation. Yes, we have the advice and judgment of others who have been through the learning process, but while their wisdom and the time might be right for them, it will not necessarily be applicable to others, or doesn't build confidence in others. We must find our inner needs individually by trial and results—'error'. We must find those objectives within our selves. The gut intelligence seems to have the wisdom of the species to inform us of what is good for us, that is, if we keep in touch with our gut feelings, and serve as a 'coach' for our sensory input.

IT TAKES A LICKEN AND KEEPS ON TICKEN

There is so much conversation these days about keeping high school students in public school. We began to wonder if it really would solve anything to patch up the old system with the old worn out image of the child we have been trying to teach. We would like to think that adding more money to the system would finally produce the answer. Well, having been a part of public education since 1960, as teachers, administrators, career counselors, and members of an experimental team, we suggest that we in education begin at the beginning and start from scratch. We are faced with revisions in our attitude toward human nature just as we are faced with a basic change in our attitude toward our living environment, with the two issues going hand in hand.

While we are being forced to examine the cultural changes required by global warming, it might be prudent to add an education page to that task as well. The education offered to previous generations did not prevent global warming, so we wouldn't expect the education now offered of the present educational system to make a useful contribution to the solution of that problem. Nor will those of us from previous generations recognize and solve the foundational weaknesses of public education without a major revision in the images we have of each other; and a change in that image is not likely soon to occur.

There have been major discoveries, however, in biological fields that could have significant positive effects on educational environments and educational methodologies, which need to be and should be investigated before a lot of money is spent by anyone on any aspect of public education. That is to say, the new neurological discoveries we have previously discussed in this book, primarily in neurobiology, need to find application in the education process before we get too excited about spending money. Once we understand the significance of the research, and decide how we will incorporate it into a system, then we will need lots of financial support.

APPLICATIONS OF NEW IMAGE TO EDUCATION

It is important to recognize that our use of the Somatic Reflection Process has been to help discover disturbing past experiences for an individual, and by bringing the somatic feelings related to those disturbances to cognitive levels, the individual can modify the judgment that caused the original disturbances. We would classify the use of somatic awareness in this manner as a *curative* process; an inefficient and expensive process that will always leave many children behind. The encouragement of somatic awareness in the early education of children is designed to be a *preventive process*. Exposing children to an environment of freedom and acceptance at a very early age, the experience of self-control and self-acceptance, will establish a more permanent set of neurological pathways, and will help them stay connected to their somatic feelings, retain the natural instinctual qualities with which they were born, and utilize those somatic feelings at a cognitive level throughout a more healthy, happy life—The "Acorn will become an Oak tree".[2]

This change from a curative to a preventive learning experience has never been tried in a public school environment, to our knowledge, and needs to be studied over an extended period with careful professional supervision and evaluation. We believe that without freedom the child will only show the image he or she thinks is needed to assume to be accepted. Without the acceptance the child will withhold the trust in others that allows him or her to reveal his or her inner purpose to self and others. Without either freedom or acceptance the child will withdraw in despair. With a balance of both freedom and acceptance, the child will be able to fulfill his or her natural purpose, and reach out to others and share. Of course no one, not even the child, can predict his or her final destiny, but in an environment of *freedom* and *acceptance*, the experience will help keep him or her on course to ultimately help reveal the stuff—the master plan, the energy and the will—with which he or she is struggling to reach his or her destiny.

A comparison of our American culture and the human environments between the early 20th and the early 21st

Centuries shows a dramatic increase in the external complexities of living as families who moved from the rural farm environment to the city. Little thought was given to the affect the city environment would have on family life—what the more impersonal industrial labor markets would do to the qualities of life. This change seems to have had a deleterious effect on the family and its ability to provide the quality of caring—the needs of Freedom and Acceptance—that was available in the rural setting. Schools have not been highly successful in compensating for this loss of family environment. Today urban family life for many is consumed with financial struggles to survive, even though both parents are employed or out of the house job seeking, so the caring is often placed in the hands of unskilled workers in commercial facilities where little knowledge of early cognitive development exists. Also, since educators and other professionals have had to work with an incomplete model of the human organism, there has been no adequate basic principle to work with, that would help policy makers and care givers to develop an educational model for cultural changes.

Now, due to recent medical research, there are more accurate models to reference change to essential needs for the public schools to use with confidence. The focus of these models for educators is on the developmental learning that takes place from conception until a child is about the age of five. There is a major social quality built in to the acceptance and control model. A child, who has experienced acceptance from his family by being his natural self at home, and has practiced self-control in school to win the acceptance of his classmates, will have learned lasting social skills. With these skills in place, a child should have less difficulty adjusting to the constraints and ambiguities of puberty and beyond. The child's early experience with the acceptance/control model has the advantage of helping the neurological development of the central nervous system and the main brain, when it is in the original developmental stage. Dr. Lise Eliot is an Associate Professor in the Department of Neuroscience at the Chicago Medical School and author of books describing the latest medical research on how we are hardwired as infants and children and on how our social influences affect growth and our gender identity. Early positive experience can optimize the ability of the brain to develop pathways of a more permanent nature, in the areas of that experience.

IDEALS FOR EDUCATION

We want to apply the idea of Feeling Awareness in the education arena through teacher and parent awareness as early as birth, or even before. This may seem far-fetched, but parents and the fetus may benefit from knowledge of what future education could mean to them; to the fetus from early treatment it receives before and after birth, and to the parent allowing the child to experience Freedom in the home before starting to school. The teacher as advisor/coach can continue the same process in K-5, guiding that freedom along with the energy towards the expressed needs of the child. A dream? Yes! If nothing more than an awakening of people to the value of nourishing human instincts for a more healthy, satisfying life, for the individual and the culture, much will have been accomplished.

We have been so used to the idea of the need for externally imposed discipline of a child, that we overlook the possibility of self-discipline, as a child learns the functional limits of self-control. By learning boundaries for exercising his control out of the early experience of freedom of being its self, the child will learn to condition his own behavior in order to receive acceptance from others. Conversely, if the child gives up too much self-control just to be liked by anyone, he quickly learns that others will tend to take over the control of him and of his time and space. It seems that a balance between the two issues of freedom and control are necessary for the individual to have the most positive experience of a full life, and for an individual to be an optimum social animal. Dealing with the basic nature of man, evident when he is open to himself and "functioning freely", Dr Carl Rogers implies, that some rational directivity in human nature exists within, when he wrote in 1961 in his book *On Becoming a Person*, "We do not need to ask who will socialize him, for one of his own deepest needs is for application and communication with others. We do not need to ask who will control his aggressive impulses, for as he becomes more open to all of his impulses, his need to be liked by others and his tendency to give affection will be as strong as his impulses to strike out or to seize for himself."

The ideal 'teacher' of the 21st Century would be characterized as a professional caregiver operating his and her own business. Professional in the sense that he or she is certified in the academic subject represented, and is directly responsible to the client—the child and the child's parents. The teacher in either public or private school, ideally speaking, would be trained to manage a class of five to ten students, and provide an environment of Freedom and Acceptance as he or she presents the appropriate academic subject matter relative to client-centered interests and as primary individual projects, except where interest of the students overlap. The teacher would have an understanding and experience with somatic awareness in his and her own life so as to be alerted to behavior patterns of the clients. This ideal image is not unlike the image of a sports coach of any age group.

The ideal school of the 21st Century is a consortium of professional academic coaches organized to support professional growth, group problem solving, centralized business management, accounting, and purchasing. The goal in this arrangement is to keep the cost of education to a minimum—the cost related to the personnel who have direct contact with the clients. Individual schools would have no responsibilities to political entities with other interests. A suitable organization at a state level, with some influence over the education process, could be made up of elected representatives of the schools—a professional society of coaches. This model is borrowed from the manner in which the medical profession has become organized to furnish a variety of professional services from one site, to reduce the cost of the services, and protect the integrity of the profession. The financing of education would probably remain directly related to the local and federal taxes.

The ideal location for a school would be in a rural area where the very young children could be out of doors, where they could examine the natural life around them, where they could wander, climb trees, play together, play alone, exercise their curiosity and their bodies, and experience their playmates/classmates without close adult supervision (although adult observation is necessary for safety). This type of experience is most important beginning preschool age whose cognitive skills are developing at a rapid rate, and their motor skills involve more large muscles than small muscles.

There are other ideal models of education, including home schooling and parent run small schools. The instinctive needs of Acceptance and Control are easily met by the parent using the teacher-coach methods if they are employing a student centered learning approach. Parents ideally act as the main teacher, much as the public school ideal of the teacher as coach, along with employed tutors in subjects that are of interest to the child but not within the knowledge skill range of the parent to act as teacher. The teacher acts as the primary facilitator of the child's education. A student-centered approach, as was amply described in *How Children Learn* by educator John Holt in the late '60s, is followed when the parent-teacher keenly observes the natural interests of the child and presents the curriculum content as a natural extension of the child's interests, giving the child the choice and responsibility for his and her own learning. We have observed that this method both serves to greatly inspire enjoyment of learning and curiosity of learning. This approach ideally holds control of one's feelings as a keynote in the learning process and has generally been known to have very positive results. The methods used in this approach ideally provide a chance for the child to feel true acceptance from his or her parent teacher-coaches as the child's feelings are always considered in the process, rather than a set and standardized curriculum presented to every child regardless of interest. And it is ideal in that it is an opportunity for communication and interchange of feelings on a daily basis between parent-teacher and the child. The home school child will ideally need to include in his and her daily schooling life a variety of experiences outside of the home to enjoy others outside of the family. These are all activities the child expresses and holds an interest in and may include such activities as sports clubs and other sports activities, small classes of all kinds at community centers and for high school age at the local junior college, activities with other children being tutored in the same subjects by the child's tutors, play days at the park and arranged field trips with other home schooled families. We have personally observed that the home school child has an opportunity, when parent-coaches follow these ideals, to interact with all ages of people, rather than only his and her own age as in a more standard school setting, and thus becomes highly socialized.

Standardized learning curriculums for public education and learning approaches may seem more economical to society in the short run and therefore more ideal for the public pocketbook that supports them (and surely this is the reason standardization in education has been far more popular these past few decades than individual student-centered approaches). But revisiting some of the ideals from the educators of the '60s and '70s with student-centered approaches coupled with ideals centered around more recent knowledge of instinctual needs and the two brain centers may provide successful innovations of our modern schools, which are now failing many students. These are ideals that support the importance of caring for the inner needs of the child and will ultimately lead them toward a healthy, creative, and successful adult life that also, in the long run, supports the overall interest of society at large.

LETTER ON EDUCATION TO PRESIDENT OBAMA

The letter that follows on the next few pages was sent from Robert Sterling to President Obama in February of 2009 and a copy was also sent to Dr. Arne Duncan, US Secretary of Education. It is lengthy but well worth the time to read as it explains the importance of including the education of our enteric nervous system—the gut—in the educational process and how to learn to keep in touch with it to inform us of what we are doing to ourselves and to make healthy decisions. The initial response to this letter from Secretary Duncan was quite positive and we were invited to attend an open conversation on education that he held in Miami a few months later. As we were not able to attend this conversation, we are still seeking further communication with the White House asking for quality rather than quantity changes in educational programs and policies for our children.

February 6, 2009

Keystone Heights, Florida

Mr. Barack H. Obama, President of the United States
of America and Family

1600 Pennsylvania Avenue NW

Washington D. C. 20500

www.whitehouse.gov

Dear Mr. President:

I have listened to you speaking on many occasions
over the past several years, and have been impressed
with your ability to use feedback from your internal
gut feelings as you speak. This ability seems to
provide you with a more accurate awareness of
human feeling relative to the logical thinking
experience toward which you focus your cognitive
attention. This holistic quality of perception and
judgment seems to have a universal appeal to people
of all cultures regardless of language. I think you call
it the "Aloha Spirit".

This simultaneous connecting of thinking and inner feeling processes working in harmony seems to communicate to others, a transparency of the integrated Self. This ability to present a combined intelligence about an issue is to me a sign that not only a harmony exists between your outside world and your inner (gut) feelings, but also it communicates a message of genuine commitment of your human nature to others. Even though others may not have achieved thinking/inner-feeling coordination, they seem to recognize a skill-a social intimacy-for that which all human nature seems to strive, and tend to reach back to the source with hope and respect. "Yes We Can".

It is rare to find a person who has developed a well-coordinated thinking/inner-feeling skill. Each one of us has the potential to develop that skill, and it is best learned at a very young age at home, in preschool and practiced throughout life. Most children do not now have that good fortune either at home or at school. Not because it is, absent from their genetic makeup, but because of cultural attitudes of distrust of human instincts. This distrust has gradually caused many natural human qualities to sink into the depths of awareness only to become a disturbance, when, if nurtured, they could become the main stabilizing force of the individual and the culture. The appreciated gut, with its instinctive power, seems to have the intelligence to modify behavior, by adjusting energy made available, when the life is being filled or being emptied. There are other constant signals from gut, but unless the digestive system is under duress and malfunctioning, the signals can be drowned out with unnecessary 'back-ground noise' from what is received from the senses. We feel of stomach ache, hunger, satiation, 'butterflies', anxiety, toilet functions, etc., but unless the signals are strong enough to overwhelm the upper brain, we have learned to ignore the gut signals and assume that the gut will take care of itself automatically-we just need to feed or empty it.

The education process required to develop a functional thinking/inner-feeling awareness seems to require greater individual freedom and acceptance than that to which most of us are accustomed. We allow the newborn early to develop his upper brain with unconditional parental acceptance, and encourage it to be free to demonstrate its instinctive skills. But by the time the child enters school, freedom to exercise instincts, with acceptance to be itself, has already been compromised. By the time the child emerges from high school, if he or she remains in school, the child has stumbled through puberty with only the shreds of the Self, remaining in his or her awareness. Some of the damage is repairable if help is available. Prevention, however, would seem prudent, for prevention covers all corners of any society in which persons may live, and like any other health issue, prevention is much cheaper than a cure.

Conception provides us with a plan for a highly complex electro-chemical operating system with intricate instructions, the DNA and RNA, for the design and construction of a future organism-a human embryo-to be born within a fixed time and with only the potential to become an independent human being. A fully functioning human brain must wait for sensory input from the outside world to utilize the neuron pool prepared during the pre-birth construction. A simplistic image of a newborn baby is a body with a functional internal energy generator with its complex nervous system, which monitors, manages, and records the internal organic operations of the organism. And, it has a nearly empty brain cavity, which gradually develops and records information from its external environments through experiences with its developing senses. The gut concerns itself primarily with what goes on inside the body, and the developing brain concerns itself with what goes on outside the body. The digestive system is of parental design at birth, and the main brain gets its growth from sensory experience throughout its life.

The DNA/RNA is the instructions for what each of us is physically designed to become. It is the architectural plan for the organic qualities of a human being with the flexibility to develop unique cognitive characteristics of its own, referenced to that plan. We all belong to the same family, but we do not look alike. We all have the same basic operating system, but we all carry out individual life experiments. We all have the same sensory equipment-sight, hearing, smell, taste and touch; but we tend to perceive the same things differently. It would seem that our major differences begin to appear as we begin to meet the outside world of diverse environments. This combination of circumstances over which there seems to have been no external determinants, except for the chancy attraction of the two genders, must rely on both its instincts and its experiences to continue its cognitive development after birth. We seem to be stuck with the luck of the draw, yet we are expected to find our own way into, and to express our own uniqueness in those environments.

This condition of only luck would be true if it was not for the guidance of the operating instincts with which we were born. This gut intelligence, perfected over eons of time, seems not just for use during the early post birth years. Nature is not wasteful with energy or experience, it rarely throws anything away that is useful, but seems to conserve and build on what works, and recycles that which does not work. In order for the enteric nervous system-the gut-to inform us of what we are doing to ourselves, we need to learn how to keep in touch with it and to use it. If we do not use it, we are likely to lose it and lose our way in life.

Educators seem to have the task of offering information for both the alikeness and the uniqueness, and seem to have done a fair job of presentation of common cognitive intelligence-what those in our environment want us to know. What we seen to have missed is the individuality, which can only come from the inner needs of the person. Without individual freedom, a person will only show us the image he or she thinks he or she needs to assume, to be accepted. Without the intimacy of positive attention and acceptance from us, the person will withhold trust; trust that would allow him or her to reveal his or her inner purpose. Without either freedom or acceptance, he or she will withdraw from us in despair.

With a balance of both freedom and acceptance, the person's holistic life experience will be more transparent and fulfilling to him or her, for his or her self concept will be more positive; he or she will show more willingness to compromise and adapt, will demonstrate greater patience, will have energy to share, and will learn to recognize and practice ethical behavior in his or her interpersonal relationships. In an environment of freedom and acceptance, parents, educators, coaches, friends, all can help keep the student on course to ultimately reveal the stuff, the master plan, the will, and the energy with which he or she struggles to reach his or her complete humanity.

Without the balance of freedom and acceptance there is depression, lack of energy, radical judgment and the tendency to strike out and grab with little or no ability to exercise self-control.

If we look back to the 1970s, at the variety of disturbances, which were affecting the lives of people; then look at the present cultural problems generating disturbances in the lives of the present culture, we may find evidence of the same source and the same center of the problems. It may be that the differences in attitudes about the causes and effects of what is happening are related in some way, perhaps to our inhumanity, a deep long term neglect of essential inner-human need. It may be that the solution to the wide variety of disturbances, that plague us now, are a replay of what was happening back in the '60s and '70s, but was never understood and corrected. Let us look and see what we found!

It was fortunate for us to have faced the symptoms of the need for changes in how to deal with the human mind in the 1970s. While working with a licensed School Psychologist colleague, Char Smith, in a community college, we accepted the tasks of teaching and operating a Career Guidance and

Assessment Program (Career GAP). Char had experienced the impact of growing up in the 1960s in Mississippi, and I was born in Northern Ohio, carrying the direct impact of WWII in Europe, with an Electrical Engineering degree, a Masters in Religious Education, and Industrial experience in Electronics.

The convergence of these two personalities and traumas enabled us to critically look at and question what was happening in counseling methodology, particularly when we faced high school dropouts, post high school students with deficient academic skills for college entrance, students recovering from drug addiction and Viet Nan Veterans who were carrying the physical and psychological impact of war experience. The result was, the awareness that there had to be a universal, deeper level of meaning to trauma than just the details of individual's experience or awareness of only emotional-feelings. At deeper levels of awareness, we found the impact of experiences as they related to the value to the organism's life-to its internal purpose-not the sensory status of the organism to its outside environments. Something deep inside had been affected when either positive of negative experience had occurred. The differences seem to be in the intensity of the experience, not in the nature of the experience. We concluded that we were dealing with the lasting impact of experience on the organism-on the design objectives of the organism whatever that design could be.

After many hours of counseling, reflecting on the feeling experiences with individuals and groups, bypassing, as much as possible, the details of the individual disturbances, we located a center of intelligence in each individual's cognitive awareness, that could compare memorable details with gut feelings about the same happening. We then let the person reassess his own meaning of the experience and gain a new perspective-a new fresh image of the Self. We found that the experience of following the present feeling of disturbance back through time to the first instance-the memory of the first awareness, we could reach a source of information that seemed to have a record of the impact of the trauma or satisfaction on the organism. There seemed to be an important level of intelligence deep in stomach area that, if contacted, could provide feedback to inform the cognitive center—the upper brain—of the needs of the organism on a continuous basis. We reflected with each other in the same manner. We finally found that our experience validated what students were teaching us, and from that we were able to develop a methodology for the process by which an individual could work with himself.

At the time, we had no idea of the physiology involved. It was not until 2004; while Char was working on her Masters thesis, that she found the neurological research that seemed to validate our findings in the '70s. When she introduced the research results to me, the early clinical experience immediately took on a new life for me.

I, we perhaps, would be most interested in volunteering time, with some level of your education staff, presenting new material relative to K-12 education. The concepts I have sketched are based on life experience, diverse education, teaching, coaching, and counseling experience, new medical research, and a lifetime of tangential experimentation. The form of the recorded material in support of these concepts consists of published and unpublished articles by my colleague and I, from 1972 to the present.

References:

Eliot, Lise, PhD, (1999). *What's Going On In There? How the Brain and Mind Develop in the First Five Years of Life.* New York, NY: Bantam Books.

Gershon, Michael D., M. D., (1998). *The Second Brain: Your Gut Has a Mind of Its Own*, New York, NY: Harper Collins.

Love, S., M.A., MA, PMA. (2007). Using Somatic Awareness as a Guide for Making Healthy Life Choices. In *Somatics Magazine-Journal Of The Mind/Body Arts and Sciences*, Volume XV, Number 2.

Love, S., M.A., MA, PMA. (2008). Healing the Trauma of the Body/Mind Split through Accessing Instinctual Gut Feelings. A Protocol for Facilitating the Somatic Reflection Process (SRP). In *Somatics*

Magazine-Journal of The Mind/Body Arts and Sciences, Volume XV, Number 4.

Sincerely,

R.W. (Bob) Sterling

sterlingrwalter@gmail.com

cc Dr. Arne Duncan, Secretary of Education

FARM TO FACTORY

More needs to be said—much more—about the *Body-Mind Split* to which is referred in the letter to President Obama. That letter focused on the problems of education, only one of the many cultural changes to be made when he took office. But since education seems to be fundamental to other cultural changes, and little has been discussed or published about applying recent experience and medical research to education curricula, we wanted to share the human image now defined by the second intelligence center in the gut.

There is and has been a lack of Will to make changes of any sort, simply because of a lack of a clear image of human nature. None of us live long enough to form a clear picture of how cultural trends affect the minds and bodies of human beings—all life, and the planet as well. Even if we had possessed the longevity to do so, it would have been useless without the conscious "wisdom of the ages", each of us has had stored in our DNA/RNA. To develop a positive image of the gut without modern scientific enquiry and without modern materials and technology could never have been possible. Just how long, and for how many generations, has anyone been aware enough to access this gut wisdom and to have consciously achieved a direction toward their goals throughout their lifetime? The enteric nervous system has been used subconsciously, but the image of this intelligence has generally been one of interference rather than in support of successful human behavior.

It may seem trivial, but much of the world's culture has moved from an Agricultural Based environment to a Industrial Based environment, assuming that the human mind and body would successfully adapt without giving the affect on human nature much thought. One of the issues in play during the transition from Farm to Factory and city life has been the lack of conscious concern for human nature—and all nature as well. The change-makers had their religion to reward them in the hereafter with money in the bank. Still another factor involved over this entire span of time was the promise of an easier, more comfortable way of life. The simplistic image of human need was "bread and butter on the table," and a "roof over their heads." Few if any of the change-makers had the remotest dream that there might be a positive neurological relationship between the human mind and body. Change took place with ignorance and misuse of the gut intelligence, not with consciousness of the instinctual need for human freedom and acceptance. Much seems to have been lost in this cultural change, and among the most crucial lost was time for reflection—quiet time—supported by the lower 'noise' level, i.e., the sounds of nature. Education was a process designed to teach factory and social skills in order to produce factory workers and 'good citizens'—the necessary accommodations to the industrial based economy.

Unfortunately, those of us who bought into these mis-representations in the past have found it very difficult to convince others to accept and apply what science has recently discovered, even when we feel physical discomfort as we become aware of it. As we have already discussed, we have found that the Somatic Reflection Process (SRP), used in the discovery of the impact of experience on the enteric nervous system as well as the central nervous system, has helped persons find a new image of themselves and a useful relationship between cognitive awareness of the Upper Brain and the inner feeling awareness of the Second Brain or the gut brain, which is also a discovery by the recent medical research of Dr. Gershon and his research team at Columbia University Medical School. We believe that the change will slowly come through experience, a more accurate image of human nature, a better understanding of the importance of environmental quality to human needs, and the early education of children centered on becoming aware of their human instinctual needs.

THE ANALOG OF DISCOVERY

When examining how we learn, educate our species, discover new innovations, and continue as a species, it might be useful for us to reflect together over the past hundred years to think and feel what we humans have accomplished with our collective intuitions for our world of environments and our inner human need's domain. This will be a valid and useful reflection if we use the new image rather than the old. We need to experience our gut-reaction as we look for human inner needs satisfaction from the environments of the outside world.

As humans, we have the internal power of nature to use our own capacity to think, feel, and learn. In the past we have had little knowledge of the gut beyond its digestive function, and only recently have we begun to improve our understanding of that function. We, as individuals, have lost conscious contact or strayed from the conscious use of internal instinctual human functions.

Dr Gershon's research has discovered the ENS of the gut as a major source of dependable influence on decisions of genuine inner needs of the organism, and the ENS can be viewed, as the result of his research, as having a substantial part in the mental and physical health of the person. Because of the cultural effort to promote the upper brain—and the heart—as the centers of intelligence, and denigrate the instinctual intelligence of the inner body, we tend to operate around the less reliable central nervous system in our daily lives, and get lost from our genuine human needs, which are located primarily in the enteric nervous system in the gut. Fortunately, the ENS is constantly operating even though we pay little conscious attention to it, until we are hungry, or it malfunctions—then we at least know its there. The ENS doesn't seem to care what we think or dream about it, as long as we feed it, pay attention to its needs, and do not interfere with its functions. However, the gut makes no promise of the quality of health and behavior of an organism, to an outside force that interferes with the very nature of its experimental success.

There is a useful analogy that we ran across not to long ago, which demonstrates a human need for an intuitive skill. This simple example utilizes a path through a forest to describe the human path through life. The more we use the path to get through the forest the more we depend on that path to get to the other side. Without warning, a tree fell across the path making it impossible to use the old path, requiring a new one be cut through to the other side. While a disturbing challenge, by thinking and feeling our way along step-by-step we can make a new path, which solves the passage problem and serves our instinctual need of self-control. So, when we face a seemingly impossible problem before us, maybe we need to use our built-in intuitive skills to find a new path to change our thinking to satisfy inner needs. This same analogy can serve in dealing with both human and non-human problems.

This leads us to the concept of human instinctual need. In the early days of animal life we are told that the ancient 'snake' brain was programmed for security of the animal—a matter of life or death which could be decided as a matter of "fight or flee." Moreover, the present gut brain contains remnants of this program, which seem to have adapted to the solution of other more complex problems of decision-making for the human organism. This seems to have become part of the feeling content of intuition—especially concerning matters of danger to the gut itself. But also in the technical sense when examining the possibility of a solution to a technical problem, a small voice will come from an inner source: "That idea will not work" or "That will work"! And, there may not be an immediate clear explanation for this often, correct signal.

In the field of electronic, industrial product-development, intuitive skills are constantly challenged to provide less expensive solutions to problems which are built-in and worked in the research phase of the product. In order to meet design specifications, and cost of the product to the consumer in the manufacturing phase, this intuitive demand becomes a constant process of trial and results. The point of bringing technology into this discussion is that this human ability to intuit-think, feel, and learn, is the analog or paradigm of discovery necessary for moving from the present into the future. It is a process often miss-given to creativity rather than discovery. We do not typically see animal life, including humans, as creators, for human intelligence is utilizing only the qualities given to the species through the experience!

Nature creates the situations called problems and man discovers the solutions.

PUBERTY AND INSTINCTUAL NEEDS AFFECTING THE LEARNING PROCESS

Le piece de resistance of our idea of freedom and acceptance, to experience and develop instinctive strength in the education process of early childhood is to establish a positive self- image for youth entering the most difficult time of their life—the stretch of time between the ages of ten and eighteen when the rush of sexual hormones amplify every negative experience a child has ever had. This hazing process during puberty may be nature's way of pre-sorting of the fittest for survival. Certainly the experience would seem to have some intelligent rationale for being. On the other hand, in our modern societies, we have no way of knowing, for we have seldom if ever made preparation for the majority of youth to consider puberty as a normal open process, through which everyone has to pass. We have never defined the process of puberty with its emerging sexual maturity in positive terms that would allow us to change our view of it and to reduce the stress upon the individual that it inflicts.

The following reflections are from an actual counseling session with an individual taken from our work in the 1970s, to demonstrate a typical problem for a young women reflecting with somatic feelings experienced at puberty. This session with an adult female follows a session, in which has been revealed some clarification of highly personal issues concerning early family relationships experienced during early childhood.

The following reflections (excerpt from Smith & Sterling, 1976),[3] are focused on the time of approaching puberty when the person had not been exposed in early childhood to a conscious awareness of her somatic feelings.

Facilitator: Are there any other feelings that come in at that time?

Reflector: I think...I think I began coming aware that...they were...there were some things that...I couldn't share with them [mother and father].

F: There were some feelings that weren't open to your parents?

R: Right! There were some feelings...more physical.

F: Yes?

R: I had free time from them, and I wasn't really doing anything that they would disagree with.

F: Can you tell me the feelings?

R: It was a feeling that I wasn't supposed to need anyone anymore. I was to go out and be independent. I really did feel alone. It was compounded because there began to be things...I couldn't share with my mother.

F: What feelings couldn't be shared with your mother?

R: My feelings, I couldn't share...

F: Were your sure your feelings were alright to have?

R: No! If I were sure, I would have shared them.

F: You were left alone to feel different...separated from your parents by those feelings? Did you feel like the only one who ever had those feelings?

R: No! Just a minute...stop asking questions and let me get to those feelings!

...........................longpause................

I still keep coming up with what I came up with before.

F: Go ahead...bring it up again...it's ok.

R: It just seemed like...it's a sexual thing.

F: Let's have it!

R: Well, that's it...that's what I mean...the sexual feelings I had..............I didn't have any sexual feelings except that I wanted to be close to...and I...

F: You weren't supposed to be close to anybody?

R: I was supposed to wait to need anybody...until the proper time...but I did and I put myself down for needing anybody in any way. I struggled with that all through high school.

F: Is the basic feeling at all like the feelings back when you were a little younger...alone, empty ...isolated...does that feel the same?

R: Yes!

F: And how were you dealing with those feelings in high school?

R: Experimenting underground.

F: Not able to share with anyone?

R: No!.............

F: You felt pretty scared?

R: Uh......huh

F: Alone most of the time, and empty?

R: Guilty!

F: Let's look at the basic feelings...does anyone support your feelings as a person during that time?

R: Attention from boys.

F: Does that attention you received from boys support your feelings as a person? Does it help your aloneness and emptiness?

R: No!

F: Was there anyone that you could share your feelings with?

R: I had one friend...we could talk about whatever we felt like talking about.

F: About your basic needs...your gut feelings?

R: No, not really.

F: About, how to get close to people?

R: It wasn't a question of how...it was whether I should or shouldn't.

F: You weren't supposed to have a need to be close to people?

R: I was supposed to control it.

F: The need for people?

R: Yeah!

F: Could you be more specific about being close?

R: Well, I mean physically.

F: How did it feel trying to manage your feelings?

R: Confused.

F: Can you put yourself back in that time and find the gut feelings?

(Pause).....empty...really alone! I needed somebody. You know, my friend and I didn't

really share our feelings...I never told her I felt alone and empty...or even guilty and afraid. I really didn't tell her any of my feelings.

F: You compared details of your lives?

R: Yeah! That's all.

F: Can you now go back to your feelings and discover what you were looking for?

R: (Pause)......I needed somebody to accept me and care about me—I needed someone to share my feelings with, that would understand. Yeah I think that's what I wanted all the time...to feel accepted by someone for what I was inside.

F: Your feelings?

R: Yeah!

F: How did this reflection feel?

You mean, what we just did?

F: Yes. Do you feel accepted?

R: Yes! It feels really good. I have never done this before. In fact, I don't think I have ever really shared my feelings with anyone before.

F: What have you learned about yourself from these reflections?

R: (Pause)...I've lived under a lot of judgments...and I tried to please everybody and myself at the same time. I found out that I couldn't do that. In a way, I'm still dealing with all of it...I still have the judgments. At least now, I can understand better what I'm dealing with.

F: In the present?

R: Yes, I feel better about myself.

> *F: Can you now define the main issues in your life?*
>
> *R: I think,....I've always needed acceptance for doing what seemed necessary for me to do*

It was revealed in an earlier session that this person built her self-concept on a persona of performing in a manner that pleased her parents. She offered this information in a review of her childhood experience with these words:

> *"I have often been aware of responses that I have made to situations and people that did not serve me as a person—did not fill me. I find my Self in the middle of such responses understanding logically why I respond, as I do to the details of the experience but also aware that my responses make no sense from an inner feeling point of view. When I experience my Self responding over and over again without any consideration for my inner needs, I feel unacceptable as I am naturally, guilty that I have to pretend that I'm something I'm not, afraid that I'll always have to pretend, and angry that I've trapped my-self. It feels hopeless in my emptiness that it will never change. In this state of emptiness I try to hide the awareness of my inner feelings, thinking that no one can accept me if they know how I really feel inside".[4]*

Later in the session she volunteered:

> *"This dilemma continues on in time until I produce crises that force me to disclose my discomfort to anyone. It is in moments of crisis that I openly begin to take the responsibility for feelings I have hidden for years. At puberty, I was set up to rebel against external authorities and got trapped in that rebellion. The set up to rebel developed from my loss of spontaneous feelings of early childhood to external*

judgments of authorities. It was my perception that I needed to follow these external judgments- give away the control in order to be accepted. The implication of such a perception, that I needed to give my natural Self away to authorities, was the judgment that my instinctive feelings could not be trusted to get me the acceptance of the authorities—of anyone. The rolls I assumed, to take the place of the directions provided by my inner feelings, proved to be empty. I know I had some awareness of my emptiness but up until puberty, my awareness was not evident enough to be convincing-that the rolls didn't work. Prior to puberty, I thought that I simply needed to get better at playing the roles to gain acceptance, These roles I had taken on to control my inner feeling responses, seemed too be a demand to perform in order to be acceptable. The trap, then, is that since early childhood I pretended to be something I wasn't, and at puberty there was no way to continue to consciously pretend. My sexual feelings at puberty shattered the myth that I could play a role and control my instinctual feelings. "[5]

The intensity of this typical experience seems to center on the force exerted on the nervous systems by the hormonal changes in the body at puberty. A child who has had to assume an early role to gain acceptance, had to give the control of his time and space to an overwhelming authority, and has had to hide his or her somatic feelings, from early childhood up to the time of puberty, will have developed deep habits of uncontrollable anger. If with this anger, the person doesn't realize the meaning of what has happened during childhood, and then consciously change the self-image, the experience of intimacy will never be available-having no respect for the Self; there will be no respect for others.

Freedom to be ones Self is a challenge to the mind-set of most societies, but even in the last half of the nineteenth century, psychologist like Carl Rogers recognized the basic nature of the human organism to have balancing needs in his intimate relationships with his fellow men and women. He had this to say, " We have no need to ask who will socialize him, for one of his own deepest needs is for application and communication with others…We do not need to ask who will control his aggressive impulses; for as he becomes more open to all of his impulses, his need to be liked by others and his tendency to give affection will be as strong as his impulses to strike out or to seize for himself".[6]

Is there anything a teacher, parent or the child can do to relieve some of the pressure of puberty? Dr. Eliot suggests that the self concept is served by being involved in some social activity that establishes an interest of the child, by the age of ten, which provides an important identity—a social sense of acceptance from peers—that divides his attention between his inner self and the outside world of friends. This can have the functional value for the child of producing a balance between control and acceptance, and fortify his instinctual needs from parents and peers to avoid the feeling of emptiness. There are a number of intellectual activities to suggest: music, both instrumental and vocal; art, painting, sketching, or drawing; gardening, flowers, scrubs, or trees; farming projects; animal projects; construction projects; business activities; cooking, karate, archery; whatever the child's choice and lasting interest may be. The child must invest the energy, the coach, mother, father, grandmother, grandfather, etc, must invest the attention of acceptance for support of the activity.

INCARCERATION: A NEW RECLAMATION PROJECT OF HUMAN LIFE

While we are on the subject of education, a word needs to be said here about incarceration and adult education of emotional intelligence. While we are proposing ways to prepare preschool children with positive images of themselves and to use their energy in the educational process and later life, we can identify the School of Incarceration that can have the same affects on human nature in adults, and, which is now locked-up, in useless ways, absorbing rather than contributing energy at the culture's expense. Such a project would utilize the curative aspects of the Somatic Reflection Process (SRP) on feeling, which was the door opened to us in the 1970s.

The rehabilitation of these men and women is simplified by the very fact that they are gathered in the same place, and many would be eager to have a chance to regain their self-control and become accepted in society. As in the early pre-school program for the children, by the time these adults meet the stresses of society once again they would have had, through participation in a reclamation project we are proposing with the Somatic Reflection Process as a center piece learning process, the experience of dealing with each other around the principles of balance of inner and external need satisfaction. This project would also provide opportunity for validation of the methodology under the most severe pressures to be found in society.

There seems to be a strong correlation between PTSD from earlier life experiences and incarcerated populations (among incarcerated populations, some studies have reported to show that PTSD has been found in over 40% of female incoming inmates and 30% of male incoming inmates). With the possibility that a third or more of people imprisoned initially are suffering from a severe stress-related illness, the use of the Somatic Reflection Process to offer all individuals who are incarcerated into a self-awareness educational experience, seems like an obvious step in the right direction for both the prison and after-prison-life experience in order to yield a higher quality of life, with less undesirable incidents of behavior, and thus being cost effective to society.

Presently, we have a more military model of prisons than an educational one and the emphasis is on changing the behavior of the individual rather than exploring the root cause of the behavior. We see this present system as over spending and failing to work—both failing to serve the needs of the individual and of society. One only has to look at the statistics to see that our emphasis on behavior rather than feelings and learning who we are and what we need as human beings is failing us. We could turn these penal institutions into learning living communities that train both the head and gut instinctual feeling brains and, if it worked, the results could turn our society toward prosperity and good emotional health.

As long as our institutions, both educational and penal, for both children and adults, continue, at best, to train our thinking brains and exclude our awareness of our instinctual second brain, we will lack the emotional intelligence needed to advance toward benevolent evolution of the human species.

CONCLUSIONS

The doctrine of "original sin" has been used by many church organizations, as the basis for distrust of human instincts. This doctrine was a product of the Roman Church during the time of organization and doctrinal formation of the church, and was by no means universally accepted. A fellow in the 4th Century by the name of Ambrose proposed the idea, and down through the centuries denominations have accepted his idea that human instincts are unreliable. The idea is that we are "… descendents of Adam, and, therefore, have inherited the sins of Adam". The churches that perform the rite of baptism are acknowledging the doctrine, and are performing this rite to "wash that sin away". These same mind-sets are still prevalent in many parts of the world and are still ignoring the damaging effects of this attitude on human experience. With the recent research in neurobiology of our genetic makeup, the DNA and RNA, and the similarity of the DNA in all life, it is quite apparent to us that we need to take a long look at what we are doing to our selves. We expect other forms of life to become what they were designed to be—the Acorn—and it can only become an Oak Tree—but we are still fearful to let the human animal become what it is designed to be. We seem willing to destroy human beings rather than risk nurturing them in Freedom and Acceptance. It is very likely that human deviant behavior is caused by the loss of contact with the somatic feelings, the instincts—the natural purpose. And, the longer the condition lasts, the more extreme the deviant behavior can become—for any human being.

It is our feeling quality that makes us as human beings each more alike than different. The main difference between "you" and "me" is the quality of the environment (experience) to which we were exposed after birth. These are significant differences, but not enough to separate us from each other, if we have learned to use our thinking and feeling skills together in our social negotiations. We are most alike in the inner body intelligence at birth, and most different in the outer intelligence of our sensory experience after birth. In other words, we each have a thinking quality of our own, and an inner feeling quality that has the same needs in every one of us, and a small unique genetic difference, the combination of which makes us unique and individual.

The issue, we think we have raised is the difficulty in combining the thinking and feeling dimensions of our human organism to balance the use of the upper brain with its central nervous system in such a manner that the upper brain will not interfere with and/or damage the use of the gut brain with its enteric nervous system. It is, after all, the ancient brain with its enteric nervous system that provides the stabilizing influence of functional intelligence of the human organism.

There is a much larger picture to be painted from turning our attention inward—which comes from our reflecting on the workings of our nature. It is the harmonious strength of what we find in human nature, as long as nature in all its forms is the 'hitching post' of our mobility, adaptability, and our intuition; and as long as we are willing to take a critical look at our inner feelings and learn from our experiences of life. But there is an infinite world we are in that is also nature, a nature that sustains us, a nature that created us, a nature that we need to understand both from the perspective of the telescope and the microscope.

We are immediately faced with a duality of looking outwardly and inwardly, just as has been found through the examination of the human anatomy. The first immediate aspect of nature, which grabs our outward-attention, is massive harmonious mobility, everything moving as a unit, but with a flexibility that implies an adaptability, which keeps the system together as a unit in spite of minor changes. Our intuition can postulate that there is a pervasive type of intelligence that seems to be in control, which can bring a harmonious form of life out of chaos. Is it possible that the nature of everything on the earth, on which we live has been established by the nature of the universe—by way of accidents—capable of bringing its materials together to form divers types of order out of chaos.

Coupling the findings of the early clinical studies we have presented and the findings by Dr. Michael Gershon, we can postulate that our instinctual needs of acceptance and control are not only giving signals in our body of their existence (emptiness and fullness in the gut area), but are also directly affecting the communication between the enteric nervous system and the upper brain. Our clinical studies have demonstrated that feeling acceptance and feeling in control of one's own responses are two instinctual needs of the human being. We can accept this and understand that people have these needs and feelings, and can build a new educational system based on this assumption or we can go on ignoring these findings and keep the old failing system of primarily educating the upper brain, producing a disastrous splitting of body/mind awareness. If we accept this understanding and importance of the relationship of the two instincts of acceptance and control of one's on responses and the gut brain of human beings, we must educate not only the upper brain, but also our awareness of our instinctual feelings in our gut region. We are then compelled to give respect to the gut brain and gut feelings of emptiness and fullness as informing us of something viable concerning our needs and direction as human beings. We now have the scientific evidence that the gut region does have responses of its own intelligence that are not dependent on the intelligence of the upper brain.

We are calling for further psychological and educational studies of the meaning of these gut responses, based on the findings of the clinical studies we have provided. It is not enough for modern psychology to keep dabbling in the discussion of gut feelings and gut intuition, without further depth study of what that precisely means and pertains to in psychological terms. Once fully understood and accepted in psychological terms, these findings will surely have direct application to the educational process.

We postulate that a major change, the turn around in our collective thinking, depends on how we educate children from birth through elementary school and beyond. We can assist young children to continue to develop constructive use of their instincts, to freely use their gut feelings, free from damaging external judgments early in life. We postulate that if we can accomplish a simple but difficult change in perspective, children will furnish the energy, the desire to learn what they need to know and when they need to know it. According to their unique design, they will become more self-disciplined, more responsible, and more productive social human beings.

It is still "morning in the abdomen".

"Disease is a vital expression of the human organism."
(Dr. Greg Groddeck)

CHAPTER ELEVEN:

THE NEW IMAGE OF HUMAN NATURE AND DIS-EASE

With the new image of human nature now validated by the medical research of Dr Michael Gershon, we are better prepared to fight dis-ease than ever before. It is important that we pay attention to this new consciousness of our two centers of intelligence—two brains—so we can finally make decisions in our lives that care about the whole person, truly reduces stress in our lives, and provide the necessary levels of nutrients to feed all our needs as human beings. We now can see that we have ignored our humanness, our human nature, and this has led us to great amounts of dis-ease and discomfort. But we live on the cusp of a Renaissance in consciousness of who we truly are and we can now begin to thrive on this exciting edge of our humanity's journey toward a greater life and a more fundamentally intelligent evolution of our species.

THE VOICE OF THE GUT AND THE CURE OF DIS-EASE

It was the discovery of the extrathymic T cell in 1989 by the renowned Japanese immunologist Dr. Toru Abo and his further development of the understanding of how it works to fight disease like cancer that gave us a way to actually measure the immune system. This also opened the door to having a concrete, medical measurement of how somatic work like the Somatic Reflection Process (SRP) affects people's health; and medical science is now studying the effects of somatic practices on the immune system by measuring the T-cell count before and after a somatic practice to explore any significant changes. Could we be seeing a way to measure the effects of the voice of the gut on our health and well-being?

In recent research at the Arthur G. James Cancer Hospital and Research Institute at Ohio State,[1] immunologists have been studying the effects of a variety of stress reduction somatic techniques including breathing meditation and acupuncture. These somatic techniques have been found in their medical research to reduce stress significantly and thus have positive effects upon the immune system and the T cell count. Immunologists found through the measurement of T cell counts that ongoing psychological stress negatively affects the immune system by disrupting the communication between the nervous system, the endocrine (hormonal) system, and the immune system, thus lowering the T-cell count and the ability of the body to fight dis-ease. The stress studied is not short-lived stress but rather chronic stress over a period of time, like the type we experience caused by difficult relationships with family, friends, and co-workers, or by the ongoing stress of high performance demands interpreted by the Central Nervous System from the external world that ignores the needs of the ENS. With a high enough T-cell count, the immune system has been found to have the ability to eliminate cancer cells and restore health.

In his books *Anti-Cancer: A Way of Life* and *The Instinct to Heal*, Dr. David Servan-Schreiber cites numerous recent medical studies concluding that the ability to keep one's emotional state in balance and stress free is also important in aiding the immune system in its work to fight off alien cancer cells and tumor growth. Somatic practices that may significantly reduce stress are being studied in private practices and in clinical trails for use as adjunctive therapies for cancer patients. Some oncologists, as those in the Cancer Centers of America, that are more private and not bound to the same pharmaceutical protocols of other medical centers, already have these therapies in place, and report great success in boosting the immune system of cancer patients employing these mind-body therapies including Laughter Therapy, Music Therapy, Relaxation Therapy, Art Therapy, deep breathing and meditation, yoga, guided imagery, and other complementary alternative techniques, along with the traditional medical approach.

Due to the significant part that the immune system plays in the prevention and occurrence of cancer, current medical thought is that it is of major importance that people who have cancer or are at risk of cancer do everything possible in their lives to reduce the stress that potentially lowers the immune system. Reiche et al confer in 2004 in the *Lancet Oncology* that our psychological wounds set off stress responses that release cortisol, and inflammatory factors that slow down our immune system and can contribute to both the growth and spread of cancer. Of course, some tension in life is important to spark our need for activity and to help lead us to goals we set for ourselves and to pursue a healthy amount of interaction with the world around us. But the stress we do not need and that is potentially harmful to our immune system is the inner stress that is signaled by different negative emotions like guilt, shame, anger, loss and fear, which are generally caused by on-going difficult events and human relations. These emotions are signals that we are in need of attention to our inner awareness of how we feel in general and the need to look deeply into the state of our being and at our underlying feeling of emptiness in the gut region of our bodies. When we feel these difficult feelings, our energy is stuck—not flowing past these emotional feelings but rather moving in a circle and blocking the production of endorphins in the gut, where according to the findings of Dr. Gershon's medical research, 50% of all our endorphins are made. Without the ample production of endorphins, our immune system is lowered.

You may notice that when you are angry and in what we could call "a tizzy" and feeling angry or when you are feeling negative about yourself and your life and you feel like you are "in the dumps", or you are caught up in the "clutches of fear", you can not feel happy feelings in your body. In fact, in this difficult emotional state, you may describe your feeling in your gut, the major producer of endorphins necessary for the happiness state, to be at that time as a "gut knot". And that is exactly right, your gut is tied up and so are your endorphins that need to flow through your body for your immune system to function optimally. For cancer patients (and actually for all people seeking optimal health) this awareness of stress in our body is extremely important because stress keeps us from having a healthy immune system that is necessary to fight off and eliminate cancer cells in the body. Dr. Toru Abo proposes in his book *Your Immune Revolution* that the human body with a healthy immune system can fight off most diseases, including cancer cells in the body (barring the body is not overwhelmed by a toxic environment that not even the healthiest of people can endure).

Unfortunately, we have been limited as human beings in our common knowledge of methods for dealing with the stress of difficult emotions and thus often try to repress these feelings or to submerge them with ineffective methods, like too much food, alcohol, glamour, consumerism, over-working, and avoidance. At best, we may know to get busy doing things that are healthy like exercise, breathing techniques, or artistic endeavors. These healthy activities may surely help and make us feel better and may go a long way in even boosting our immune system in this stressful condition of illness. But without dealing with the root of the feelings, our ease of emotional pain is probably only temporary because the feeling issue is not really dealt with and it is just forced to lay fallow in our unconscious to wait for another moment to be triggered, arise again, and produce more stress in the future. If we are to make a garden of the mind and body that can flourish and be strong enough to fight off diseases effected by stress and a lowered immune system, we must not just nurture the top soil of our psyche, but also enrich deep into the body and soul where growth and life reaches for nourishment.

These difficult emotions like guilt, anger, and fear are signals that need to be studied by each individual and ultimately dealt with, rather than avoided or suppressed until meeting them periodically again in crisis or disease when they become yelling at us for attention so loudly that we can no longer ignore them. This is not to blame any one individual who becomes ill for not tending his or her "garden" properly, for this is not a problem produced by the individual alone nor one that a single individual has and can achieve wellness alone for themselves. This is a problem for humanity in general, a struggle in the growth of our human species that we all face together, and a struggle that must be resolved on a wide cultural level for both Eastern and Western societies, as it partially originates and involves the community in which each of us have lived in the distant past and/or is presently living. As we have pointed out in earlier chapters, our species has ignored our human nature and our human needs and this has produced sick societies. The individual who is ill from such stress is responding normally to what has been produced by the environment they live in. And the resolution of the problem for the individual will require another human being in the immediate community to give support and caring for the person's feelings in processing the repressed feelings. From what we have found in counseling, the emotional care needed from others requires more knowledge of the emotional body than most people have who are serving at this time as either family, friend, or professional caregivers. And with the growing number of caregivers needed due to the rise of illnesses in our society, this lack of emotional knowledge supports a need of somatic education for both healing and healthy development to begin in early education in our schools, as well as in adult education.

We are all made in our DNA to need each other in this process of inner discovery of our feelings and needs. We need, at least initially, another human being to communicate with and reflect with us on who we are so that we can realize our humanness and likeness as human beings. This is an instinctual need and you know this as you share your gut feelings with another person and realize the similarity of your feeling responses and the humanness that you share. It feels good and it feels like a burden and weight of stress is lifted from us when we do this.

British psychoanalyst Dr. John Bowlby's work with attachment between the infant and caregiver showed us many years ago that human babies need human touch to develop and thrive, and that we are designed by nature and instinctual need to live a shared journey with other humankind from early infancy. This need for human attachment can certainly be extended throughout all of life and the lack of this attachment is devastating for adults who have long lost the ability to trust others due to early and repeated trauma that has left them disconnected from their own internal sensations, feelings, and awareness of instinctual needs. The need for community, attachment, safety, containment, and what we might overall call Acceptance must have a high priority and primary concern in our society if we are going to have a healthy people. Illness is possibly preventable if we work together as a culture, a community, in our schools, even at the work place, and certainly as a family on a daily basis to reduce stress and to share our feelings together and care for each other. Together, we must pay attention to the feelings in our guts and attempt to communicate what the voice of the gut is telling us about our human needs. And thus due to our instinctual need for each other and the need to share our human consciousness with each other, neither the presence of nor the elimination of illness is not dependent upon just the individual who is sick but also of the culture, of our humanity, of our entire knowledge of what is necessary to be a healthy human being and a healthy humankind.

These feelings that we feel under chronic stress are not negative emotions in their usefulness, we just call them negative because they feel difficult and because they are the pain of the emotional body. But like the pain of the physical body, it is useful as a signal that something is ill in our psyche. And it is necessary to have these emotions to raise a red flag to make us aware of the condition that our emotional body is in. What we are often lacking is a method that we can use to practice listening to these emotions. Patients of stress related illnesses, and really all human beings, need a somatic method that they can rely upon to look deep within and examine what the gut emptiness and gut knots are all about— to examine what needs we are having that are not being met and how we might go about filling ourselves so that we do not have to become ill from undue stress.

Without this knowledge of a method of inner discovery, clearing, and renewal, we find ourselves conducting our lives similarly to the person driving a car until the gas gauge begins to register on empty and does not know where to drive to the nearest gas station for a fill-up. We can run out of gas too. And unfortunately our modern cultures both East and West, unlike many indigenous cultures of our ancestors, have little place for emotional healing gas stations available routinely and ritualistically for everyone to share. Where can we go to be filled up when we are aware that our emotional immune system is low? And what if we are like so many struggling people who just haven't the money to pay for counseling or a healthy somatic practice during this low emotional stage? In that emptiness, if we do not have the support and knowledge to fill ourselves up and get back in full motion on the road of life, we, like our cars, will just sit idle in a state that brings eventual deterioration to our internal system.

The problem of emotional emptiness is easy to ignore by an entire culture because emotional feelings are not tangible and are unseen even under the microscope. So, we have been under the illusion that if we just suppress these feelings or "buck up" without expressing these emotions, we can deal with life and get ourselves on the road to happiness. The rise in the frequency of illness in the last decades has proven this line of thinking inaccurate. And with the discovery of the T-cell count, the effects of our emotional health on our physical health can now be medically studied with physical data and our emotional body must be no longer regarded as completely intangible nor unrelated and without affect upon the health and wellbeing of the human body.

DISTINGUISHING THE "YOU CELLS" AND "NOT YOU CELLS"

Immunologists are beginning to understand something about the existence and need for the immune system to have its own reflection process to identify unhealthy cells that need to be eliminated. The process and intelligence of reflection of the immune system is similar to the process of inner somatic awareness that leads to the restoration of emotional health. If we look first at the reflection and identification process of the immune system itself in fighting disease and bringing wellness to the physical body, it is easy to then demonstrate how the process of the immune system has similar elements to Depth Psychology processes, including the Somatic Reflection Process, that lead us to healthfulness of the emotional body.

Dr. Toru Abo, who saved countless lives by discovering extra thymic T cells and later in 2000 that the gastric ulcer is triggered by the dominance of granulocytes in white blood cells rather than by gastric or hyper secretions (as we had thought for 100 years), also discovered in 1996 that the immune system is compromised by stress. His findings suggest that leukocytes have an increase of granulocytes when the sympathetic nervous system is dominant and an increase of lymphocytes when the parasympathetic is activated. This means that if the autonomic nervous system is stuck in sympathetic mode caused by chronic exposure to stress, the parasympathetic nervous system is not activated and lymphocytes decrease and the number of granulocytes and inflammation increases. Without the proper amount of lymphocytes that are the immune system's ability to mark foreign cells in our body, the immune system does not have a method of identifying which cells are healthy and unhealthy, which cells are and are not cancer cells to be eliminated. We could say that as long as we have chronic stress in our lives, we are at risk of being haunted with cancer cells and becoming sick because they will continue to be produced and be of sufficient strength to go unidentified and hidden in our bodies without being eliminated by our immune system.

Dr Abo found with the identification of T cells that the immune system has the ability to mark a foreign cell (cancer cell) from a cell that is normal and then eradicate the foreign cell. This has been described as finding the "you cells" and "not you cells" and getting rid of the "not you cells". T cells continually scan the surfaces of all of our cells in our body and kill those that exhibit foreign markings.[2]

We can compare this T cell function in the physical body to the necessary process of reflection in eliminating old, outdated mental tapes and complex constellation affects that occur in the emotional body. When we explore our true feelings with the Somatic Reflection Process, and we trace our feelings and gut responses back to their origin, we find that our guilt, for instance, began with an experience when we were empty and without our human instinctual needs being met. It was in that state that we may often find that we accepted the negative thinking judgment of another person about ourselves and who we are as a human being. This external judgment is foreign to the assessment of our own internal assessment of needs and may become such an automatic tape in our thinking that we do not remember where the idea came from in the first place. We may carry this external assessment of ourselves in our consciousness for a long time and not even be aware that the thinking of these thoughts about ourselves were told to us by an authority or other important person in our lives. In that case, we may feel guilty that we did something or did not do something that someone else disapproved of and now we have laid the judgment on ourselves without question. We decide to accept that we are stupid or ugly or selfish or lazy and we feel guilty and thus depressed. And all of this is not something that we originally invented, but accepted in our emptiness, as human beings are prone to do when true acceptance for who we are is not available.

These are assessments of whom we are, with an origin from an external judgment of our organism, foreign to our own thinking in origin, that we may live with for a long time without understanding that we carry something foreign in our emotional body. We can go all our entire lives without questioning our emotional complexes or what we like to call *emotional hauntings*. So our understanding of the "you" or what we truly feel about ourselves from an inner needs perspective and the "not truly you" or what we were told we are, never gets distinguished and thus the "not truly you" becomes so integrated in our thinking that we have no way to identify what is "you" and "not truly you", except in the awareness of some distant feeling in our guts where the voice is still screaming very softly of feeling emptiness and aloneness—although it is generally true if the emotions of guilt, fear, and anger exist that we are certainly not listening to our gut instincts of emptiness and fullness. In this condition, our energy is drained, our thinking becomes distorted, and our premises often consist of lies we tell ourselves that only feed into these emotional hauntings and seem to validate our low self-opinion and esteem. Without reflection on our inner gut feelings to dislodge the external, foreign thinking from our consciousness, we cling to our misconceptions of ourselves and we cannot function at an optimal healthy capacity for neither ourselves nor those we care deeply about and our stress level is high, yet often the awareness of all of this is suppressed and unconscious until a time of crisis.

Without the caring of another human being to first reflect to us acceptance and understanding, it is doubtful that anyone ever reexamines their feelings thoroughly enough to find their way home to who they are or as Dr. Carl Jung[3] suggests, sets their foot on the *individuation* process. Once initiated with this identification of who we are on a deep feeling and somatic level, the process may begin toward true emotional healing. This is something that we as psychological somatic practitioners have seen in process for decades, going back to early analysis with Depth Psychology leading us toward the process of individuation or wholeness for health and healing. But recently, in the last decade, immunologists have begun to look at this same process of identification in the physical immune system in answer to how does the white blood cell know what cell to attack and what healthy cell to leave in tact? How does the white blood cell make the distinction between the "you cell" and "not you cell"?

What excites us about Dr Abo's research is that he is finding that disease of the physical body is naturally healed by the physical immune system using a process with a notable similarity to the somatic psychological practices that are used to treat complexes of the emotional body. Somatic practitioners have long found that clearing the emotional body by using modalities like the Somatic Reflection Process, yoga, breathing meditation, and other somatic psychology processes that bring us closer to the awareness of who we truly are and release our thoughts and emotions of who we are not from our consciousness, returns the emotional body to its natural state of wellness. Dr. Abo, with his latest book now translated in English in 2007, has found that the immune system works to heal the physical body in a similar fashion, using a similar process of identifying or "tagging" what is a "not you cell" from what is a "you cell" and being given support to naturally eliminate what is "not you".

Moreover, the health of the emotional body is affected by the health of the physical body and vice-versa. There are similarities in how they both function and how they directly affect each other. This effect leads one to inquire if there is something in certain somatic and psychological interventions that not only supports the immune system but also activates its healthy processes? Based on experience with hundreds of clients, as well as our own inner experiences of using the Somatic Reflection Process (SRP) for over 40 years on a daily basis, we have found that there is experienced with this process a relief of tension/stress symptoms and a body-feeling/mind connection that feels united and connected with a result of much more energy accessible to the individual.

We could hypothesis that the greater ability you have to distinguish between "you" and "not you" affecting your emotional body and to thus return to a normal state of body-mind unity, the better the chances for longevity and a strong physical immune system that can also tag the "not you cells" from the "you cells" to fight off physical disease. A case for the vice-versa affects of the healthy physical immune system upon the emotional immune system may also be made.

There is an ancient Daoist saying in the I-Ching or the Book of Changes that reads "As above, so below" and applies here to this relationship between the emotional body-immune system and physical body-immune system, if we might for a moment separate the two. At the heart of the body-mind connection, we understand that we are but one entity, united in body, emotion, spirit, and mind. But for the sake of scientific study, it is useful to break down and identify component parts and examine them from as many angles as possible. So we might ask, if the emotional body-immune system works in a similar fashion to the physical body-immune system, what else is similar about the two systems besides the identification of and elimination of the "you" and "not you"?

Could immunologists and somatic practitioners learn something valuable from each other by engaging together in discussion and inquiry about how these two systems work and how they might be compared or if they just may be the same in source and both a function of evolved human intelligence? It is possible that the immune system (IS) may be just the RNA intelligence converted to a repair function after birth. Since the RNA is the builder of the fetus, by differentiating the cells of the body, designating and sending cells to their proper locations of the body, at the proper time. Nature would not add-on another system if it already had a successful functional system that worked—like the RNA. It would be contrary to the add-on principle of life, to abandon the RNA and start over with a new immune system.

We suggest that the immune system is a continuation of its work—original work—patching up the wear and tear of the organism it originally built. Who or what would be more likely to recognize *my cells* or *not-my-cells* after birth and throughout life of the organism than the RNA intelligence? The implication here is that our immune system is evolving through trials of use in fighting illnesses and the bombardment of our modern world toxins and that this evolution not only engages the strengthening of the body and it's T-Cell use but also our emotional intelligence and a higher awareness of our human nature and its original DNA coding as a highly self-reflective and intelligence evolving entity. In this way, we could say that all people who are fighting to strengthen the emotional immune system along with the physical immune system, for whatever reason whether it is to overcome disease or emotional pain, are doing the work to overcome the body-mind split for not just themselves but also for the healthy evolution of our entire human species.

THE SOMATIC REFLECTION PROCESS AS A MEDICAL INTERVENTION

Twentieth century medicine led with the philosophical idea of the organ system model of dis-ease and diagnosis; and this furthered increasiing specialization and breakthroughs in imaging processes, as well as complex biochemical pathway advances. However, by the end of the 20th century, systems oriented life science emerged in the forethought of modern medical thought. And with this new growing orientation toward the non-linear in both physics and medicine, physicians using an integrative, functional medicine paradigm are now struggling in science to embrace the uncertainly that goes with it. Both the doctor-patient relationship and communication is changing to utilize heuristics of a healing partnership when time and information on dis-ease are limited and when the outcome of treatment is uncertain.[4]

As an example of this new medical perspective, the Institute for Functional Medicine (IFM)[5] describes the basic principles of their integrative model as using a patient-centered rather than dis-ease-centered approach to treatment with an interest in the web-like interconnections of internal physiological factors and the identity of health as a positive vitality. This approach views the human organism as a whole with countless points of access to affect the organism and, thus, makes intervention at any one point as possibly having a beneficial influence over the entire system. For instance, increasing the T cell lymphocyte levels has been found to beneficially influence the immune system, as we previously discussed, and stress reduction can reduce the cortisol levels, reducing the risk of cancer cell growth. With this 21st Century model of medicine and healing, we have the opportunity to move toward an integrative approach that views the imbalance of the mind-body integration as one of the pathways of disease.

Besides bringing psychotherapists and other somatic practitioners on board with the medical team to apply integrative mind-body therapies, physicians embracing the integrative approach are employing some of the mind-body techniques in the doctor-patient communication and as a diagnostic tool. Successful results are being reported by physicians, particularly in finding the trigger or circumstance at the beginning point of the illness. The Institute for Functional Medicine relates a success story with a patient who had a gastrointestinal disorder. This story serves as an example of their use of a mind-body reflection technique that asks the patient to center on the feeling in her gut to find the time she did not have her "gut problem' as the patient called it and what circumstances she experienced during the first appearance of the problem. The IFM reports that the patient was able to find the experience in her past when she first started having pain in her gut region, and it began when she lied to her mother who asked her if she had been sexually abused by her father, saying that she had not. Because this was the first time that she realized the emotional origin of her dis-ease, it was considered by her medical team as an "aha" moment and insight for her that was an initial experience of healing her GI by bringing the split between her body and mind in balance.

This clinical experience is comparable to the experiences that we have had with clients using the Somatic Reflection Process to bring awareness and resolution to a current unresolved issue that was causing the person confusion, stress, lack of energy, and sometimes medical physical symptoms. One such client sticks out in our minds. A middle aged man we were both counseling in a Behavioral Science Class (BE 100), a mandatory group encounter college orientation class in the '70s at Santa Fe Community College, was complaining of low energy due to his lack of sleep. The feeling that he got in touch with around the issue was fear and he said it related to a reoccurring nightmare that was keeping him from sleeping night after night and had for some time, although it had gotten more intense since he returned to college as an adult student.

When asked to tell the dream, he began to express that he was afraid and there was a large lady in the dream that was coming toward him. After having him get in touch with how he felt as he looked at the large lady in the dream, we had him trace the feeling of fear he expressed back to an early time in his life when he felt that way before. He was surprised to find that he found a direct link in his feelings to coming home on the ship while he was serving in the Armed Forces in World War 2 and seeing the Statue of Liberty. He had an 'aha' moment as he felt the link of the fear in the dream to returning home and to our knowledge, he did not have the nightmare again. After further sessions of the Somatic Reflection Process, the body-mind connection he made opened a door of further somatic reflection in which he was able to understand the difficulties he was having dealing with the loss of the war heroes he served with and in integrating back into society as a vet with this personal loss. Many of the same issues he faced returning home after war were similar to what he was now experiencing returning to school as an adult college student. He was able to deal with these issues with far less fear and far more effectively having sorted the past from the present impact of his experiences. His vitality also returned and we often wondered if this therapy evaded further medical problems for him had this stress been allowed to continue and sleep deprivation continued.

We bring these two stories to the reader's attention in order to demonstrate how doctors who use an integrative model in the diagnostic and healing process can successfully employ the Somatic Reflection Process.

IDENTIFYING ELEMENTS OF THE SOMATIC DEPTH PROCESS FOR MEDICAL STUDY

We thought as a way to open a much needed conversation between somatic practitioners and immunologists, we would start it by offering to identify the elements of the basic psychological experience of a somatic depth process like the Somatic Reflection Process (SRP). Perhaps by understanding what is required of the emotional body to become conscious of the true self that calls from deep within our unconscious and DNA coding, through the depth process, immunologists can apply these principles to the further understanding of the workings of the physical-body immune system and how it functions. We will be able to see some correlations of similarity that are obvious and calling out for further clinical study and comparisons using the T-cell count as an evaluation measurement in future studies.

In working through some of our own issues, as well as with the people we have coached, that cause stress in life, we have used a number of depth processes including: the Somatic Reflection Process, dream work technique processes, art as a depth process, memoir, active imagination, and authentic and somatic movement processes. In using all of these processes together in succession on a specific issue, we identified six phases of awareness that the individual might experience on the road to a deeper self-awareness and emotional healing. These are not all of the processes by any means that could be used to experience these six phases that lead to individuation and self-awareness. We think we could safely include any other somatic process that brings us closer to the awareness of the deep unconscious, authentic Self. The important aspect of the process is that it is a somatic process, a body engaging process—that it is felt and not just thought—and that it is a depth process that reveals to us what has been hidden to our awareness in our unconsciousness of who we truly are (McCabe, personal communication, 2004). We also feel that in some way it must have a self-reflective aspect that redefines who we are in our consciousness for it to be truly a depth process.

These six phases of the somatic depth process can best be summarized in terms of their relationship to each other while taking us in the process toward reaching wholeness and the integration of the psyche. It is in the sixth stage and the integration of the psyche that we believe the immune system is boosted and the body is stabilized to a more healthy balance, capable of measurement showing an increased T-cell count and a significant improvement in the health of the patient. A clinical study evaluating the T Cell count effects of the completion of these processes and six phases could yield mathematical value to this hypothesis.

We are sharing these six phases, however, not so much for study of the overall effectiveness of a specific somatic depth process, but as a guide for immunologists and other physical scientist to break down and identify the elements of the process of healing the emotional body. It is hoped that this information may yield some further clues that show similarities to the process of the immune system in healing the physical body with that of the emotional body. The more thoroughly we understand how to heal the emotional body, the better we may understand how to heal the physical body, and vice-versa. Had we had this conversation 20 years ago between immunologists and somatic depth practitioners and psychologists, immunologists may have had the idea much earlier to look for the element in the immune system that is capable of identifying "the you cell" and "not you cell", and thus the T cell may have been recognized many years prior to its actual discovery. We have no doubt that we as somatic practitioners have just as much to learn from studying the processes of healing disease of the physical body identified by immunologists; and we too could benefit from gaining a new perspective to research our own practices.

THE SIX PHASES OF SOMATIC DEPTH PROCESS

While we had not read of his work on *initiation* prior to initially identifying these six phases of depth process, there is an interesting relationship to Henderson's (1967) three stages of initiation and these six phases. The late Dr. Joseph Henderson was a renowned psychoanalyst and author who was an early practitioner of methods developed by Carl Jung to explore cultural influences on the unconscious mind. Both Henderson's model and the one we are presenting include the idea that the process of individuation or wholeness has no actual final stage or phase, as the process will always begin again. There is also an important separation in both of these models of the consciousness of the individual from the awareness of the external world that must take place before an exploration of the inner world may truly begin. This initial separation of consciousness is necessary in the individuation process of the true self identifying and accepting the "you" from the "not you", or one's authentic self and responses from the learned and often foreign and external perception of self.

In the somatic depth process, the individual moves through a cycle of six phases of depth work beginning and ending the cycle with an initiatory experience. We identify and name these six phases *Initializing* or Opening the Doorway; *Identifying*; *Dislodging*; *Dispersing* or Going Back to the Source; *Absorbing*; and *Integrating Initiation* or Experiencing the Self. Each depth method either takes the person into the awareness of a new phase of the cycle or further into the one he or she is presently in when they begin the process. The amount of time the individual stays in each phase varies. We have found in our own personal studies of these phases that we move through a phase more quickly if we employ a variety of somatic depth methods to assist us on our journey. We have also found that the Somatic Reflection Process as a primary and sole technique employed is highly successful in the movement and completion of these six phases toward self-awareness.

In the *Initializing* or Opening the Doorway phase, we become aware of an important affect we are experiencing.

This affect is part of a complex that has been triggered from an experience in the present. In this phase, we usually feel surprised to stumble across our pain but intrigued and curious about continuing our inner exploration.

Soon after Opening the Doorway, we experience the second phase that we call *Identifying*. In this phase we become aware of the source of the affect and personality complex in our past experiences, and of the meaning and impact of those experiences on us. We become aware of the state of our organism, and the source of externalized judgments in our thinking. We learn to identify the source of the external judgments about ourselves that we accepted as a part of our own thinking. We identify the confusion that accepting these external judgments has caused us. This is similar to identifying the inner critic and the difficulties we have as a result. As we identify the source of the externalized judgments and thinking that we are still using, we become aware of the difference between it and our internal, organismic needs. We become aware of the tension that occurs between our thinking and feeling and we identify the tension of opposites that we hold within our psyche. This is often painful work but we also realize that it is healing to become aware of suffering that we have held captive deep in our unconscious for so long. It is therefore also compelling.

In the third phase, we experience *Dislodging*, in which we begin to separate the awareness of our inner feelings from our thinking. With our increased awareness of the difference between our feelings and thinking, we reevaluate our thinking and decide if it serves our own needs as a person. Our thinking and feeling awareness needs to be separated in order to embrace a more effective way of thinking that considers the importance of our instinctual feelings and somatic responses.

In the fourth phase, we experience *Dispersing* or Going Back to the Source. In this phase we imagine giving up something we originally experienced as a misconception. For example, we may give up a distorted idea about ourselves that we accepted from an authority in our life or that we assumed as a child, lacking information to make an accurate assessment.

In the fifth phase, we experience *Absorbing*. In this phase, we hold onto or keep something of value to us from the depth process experience. Here we reach a deeper level of identifying the affect involved in the issue, with greater sensory memory of the experience. We keep the insights that we have during the process work and become aware of the impact of these new insights, quite often resulting in a feeling of the numinous, or a feeling of awe and a connection with energy greater from the source of life itself. In this phase, we experience a feeling of being full in the gut area of the body as we feed ourselves enlightened consciousness, an integration of some aspects of our psyche. We may feel a spontaneous healing of some physical symptom at this point in the process.

In the final sixth phase, *Integrating Initiation* or Experiencing the Self, we experience a feeling of closure. Often we continue to experience the numinous that we had begun to feel in the absorbing phase. We feel wholeness. We feel full inside our bellies and centered with our mind and body as one, connected to all of life and its source, and open to all potentiality in the universe and our own being. After a period of rest, we feel ready to undertake another cycle of depth work, but usually on a new issue or around another hidden personality complex.

CONCLUSIONS

The first obvious similarity of the healing process of these two systems—the physical body system and the emotional body system—of the human being is the need for the foreign substance of each system to be *identified* and *dislodged*. This process seems to require some intelligence building experiences. From what we are told by immunologists, the physical-body immune system has memory T cells to identify the foreign or cancer cells (similar to *Dislodging* in phase three of somatic depth processes) and both T cells and B cells eliminate these tagged cells (similar to *Dispersing* in phase four of the somatic emotional processes).

In viewing the stages, we see that in order for the *Dislodging* to be used and *Absorbed*, the person must in phase five have a greater sensory memory of an experience before healing can begin. If we assume these correlations of structure are true in these two systems of the physical body and the emotional body, then it follows that a greater sensory memory as in phase five of the somatic emotional process would follow in the physical immune system as well. Memory T cells have their identifying ability because they are thought to have encountered antigens during a prior infection, a previous encounter with cancer, or a previous vaccination.[6] The smarter and better trained the Memory T cell, the better the immune system is at identifying and ridding itself of foreign cancer cells. In the somatic emotional process, the thinking process about oneself actually changes and becomes more focused and intelligent about who it is and who it is not. In his popular book *Emotional Intelligence*, Dr Daniel Goleman coins this phrase emotional intelligence and equates better life quality to heightened emotional intelligence and feeling awareness in the body. Is it possible that like the T memory cell of the physical immune system, we could also identify and measure an emotional memory mechanism that affects an emotional immune system and actually changes one's sense of self, our self-reflective ability and our emotional intelligence?

We are sure people could reach the six phases and complete a cycle of growth of consciousness and self-awareness using many other somatic modalities besides the Somatic Reflection Process, several of which we have employed with our selves and with our patients and students, including yoga, breathing meditations, Dr. Geri Olson's[7] doll project in making the human figure as a depth process, both individual and group dream work as in the internationally known dream tender Reverend Dr. Jeromy Taylor, Feldenkrais body work, art as therapy, and authentic movement. And while we find it helpful to suggest employing an eclectic use of somatic depth processes, we do not doubt that these six phases may be reached using even just one of these modalities in thoroughness. As we mentioned earlier, we have on numerous occasions with patients reached a significant self-awareness growth that we think took the individual through the six stages and we were only engaged in using the Somatic Reflection Process (SRP) as a single modality.

The important point is not the specific somatic modality used (we all have our favorites) but what they have in common in terms of process, healing structure, somatic awareness, and stages of consciousness awakening. These are the qualities of the experience of healing the somatic emotional immune system that can be compared with what the immunologists are studying in the qualities of the process of healing the physical immune system, and vice-versa. This comparison may well bring us closer toward wellness as a human family, as well as a further understanding of our evolutionary process of being all we can be and of our innate programming in our DNA, our true human nature.

"Behind thy thoughts and feelings, my brother, there is a mighty lord, an unknown sage—call it Self; it dwelleth in thy body, it is thy body."

(Nietzsche, 1911/1999, p. 19).

CHAPTER TWELVE:

THE NEW IMAGE: OUR GUT AS A DEPENDABLE CENTER OF REFERENCE

We have described in this book a new image of humanity and a basis for that new myth. We have also taken the liberty to utilize our combined intuitive processes to carefully examine the material on which our intuitions are based—a combination of thinking and feeling intelligence from two individuals. We have conducted a daily examining of our postulations about potential new, more responsible, behavior patterns in our own lives for the past forty years. Current events in our culture have given encouragement to the process by constantly expressing and demonstrating a need for fundamental change in decision-making patterns of thought. We believe that humans have always had the same dual intelligence of two brains, as has been recently found in medical research. We conclude therefore, from the use of the new image, that we as an extended culture have simply lost effective contact with and functional use of our second center of intelligence—the gut. We conclude that the instinctual ENS, and life, isn't going to be any better, and probably worse, until we recapture and use the conscious feeling response of that center—the reliable instinctual feeling response of the gut.

It seems difficult for most of us to focus our attention on our inner instinctual gut feelings and even more difficult to learn to communicate these feelings openly to others. But, if we can not become aware of our inner needs relative to our instinctual somatic feeling responses, our experiences in relation to other people becomes centered on what we perceive outside of our space, our own bodies, and lacks an awareness of inner feelings and thus empathy and compassion. Without the effort to discover the state of our inner human needs, we become more aware of our differences from others and feel isolated and alienated from the rest of the human family—we feel the loss of acceptance of others and the loss of control of our own natural responses.

Today, we live in highly developed cultures, both modern Eastern and Western, in which our observed behavior seems to be more important than our inner life. We have been and still are required to examine everything we feel, think, and do from the points of view of what others will think, feel or act on when they become aware of our actions. In such a field of experience, we educate our thinking—outer awareness—and leave almost totally unacceptable our inner instinctive feeling awareness. We leave our inner feeling awareness as a reliable spontaneous reference center of our inner needs to be inexperienced in its job and we let it become a covert seemingly disruptive force to ourselves and to others around us.

We may become convinced early in our experiences that our inner feelings are the weakest part of us and that decisions based upon our inner feelings were judgments that led to crisis. This means that we have learned to ignore the rational directions of our life processes, on the state of which our inner feelings report. We did this in favor of our thinking awareness that we learned to operate according to outside systems of thought. Without making the effort to go back over past experience, reflecting on our feeling awareness and reassessing the impact of each experience on ourselves, it is easy for us to remain convinced that our inner feeling center is totally unreliable—a disruptive interference and a source of aggression towards ourselves as well as others.

If we do not learn to become aware of our inner Self— our inner issues from moment to moment—and share that awareness with others, we set ourselves up to encounter a crisis of guilt and isolation in any of the many possibilities in human experience.

Our years of experience in sharing this inner awareness of ourselves with many others in reflection on our gut responses, leads us to the inevitable conclusion that this reliable center of reference is in all of us regardless of our thinking experience, and we can expect to find it in all members of the human family. It is there, often carefully maintained hidden in guilt and shame but very much alive and well. It is waiting for the encouragement of acceptance from another member of the human family to free its Self from the guilt, to take control, to make the break for freedom and be itself.

Because we do not understand the brain very well we are constantly tempted to use the latest technology as a model for trying to understand it. In my childhood we were always assured that the brain was a telephone switchboard. ('What else could it be?') I was amused to see that Sherrington, the great British neuroscientist, thought that the brain worked like a telegraph system. Freud often compared the brain to hydraulic and electro-magnetic systems. Leibniz compared it to a mill, and I am told some of the ancient Greeks thought the brain functions like a catapult. At present, obviously, the metaphor is the digital computer.

John R. Searle

AUTHORS' NOTES AND DEFINITIONS

NOTES ON REFERENCES

Chapter 3

1. The following dialog was first recorded by tape and transcribed as material for a text for classes we were teaching in Behavioral Science 100 at Santa Fe Community College, Gainesville, FL. Sterling, R.W. and Smith, M.C. (1976). *Borne of the human family*, printed at Santa Fe Community College, pp.79-84.

2. Ibid., pp. 103-108.

3. Ibid., pp. 111-113.

4. Ibid., pp.115-116.

Chapter 4

1. Campbell, J. (1976, first published 1959). *The masks of God: Primitive mythology*. New York: Penguin.

2. Eliot, Lise, (1999). *What's going on in there? How the Brain and mind develop in the first five years of life.* New York,: Bantam Books.

3. Gershon, Michael D., M. D., (1998). *The second brain: Your gut has a mind of its own*, Harper Collins.

4. Ibid., p. 17.

5. Ibid., 8-18.

Chapter 5

1. Gershon, Michael D., M. D., (1998). *The second brain: Your gut has a mind of its own.*

2. Jung, C. G. (1959). Psychological types. In V. Laszlo (Ed.), *The basic writings of C. G. Jung.* (R. F. Hull, Trans.). New York: Random House. (Original work published 1938).

3. Ibid., p. 208.

4. Ibid., p. 251.

5. Ibid., p. 229.

6. Winnicott, D. W. (1971). *Playing and reality.* New York: Penguin Books.

7. Myers, I. B. (1980). *Gifts differing.* Palo Alto, CA: Consulting Psychologist Press. Isabel Myers' book was published a couple of years after we last saw her.

8. Hillman, J. (1996). *The soul's code: In search of character and calling.* New York: Warner Books, p. 6-7.

9. Ibid., p 259.

10. Ibid.

11. Winnicott, D. W., *Playing and reality.*

12. Jung, C. G. (1969). Conscious, unconscious, and individuation. (R.F.C. Hull, Trans.). In H. Read, M. Fordham, & G. Adler (Eds.), *Collected works of C. G. Jung*

(V. 9, pp. 275-289). New York, NY: Pantheon Books, Inc., (Original work published in 1939).

13. Stein, M. (1998). *Jung's map of the soul*. Chicago: Open Court, p. 94.

14. Ibid., p. 128.

15. Ibid., p. 117.

16. Conger, J. P. (1988). *Jung and Reich: The body as shadow*. Berkeley, CA: North Atlantic Books.

17. Weis, R. (1973) *Loneliness: The experience of emotional and social isolation*. Cambridge, MA: The Massachusetts Institute of Technology. p. 22.

18. Stein, M., *Jung's map of the soul*.

19. Winnicott, D. W., *Playing and Reality*.

20. Fox, M. (1999). *Sins of the spirit, blessings of the flesh*. New York, New York: Harmony Books.

21. Gendlin, E. T. (1981). *Focusing* (2nd ed.). New York: Bantam Books, p. 35.

22. Ibid., p. 35.

23. Wittine, B. (2003). Jungian analysis and nondual wisdom. In J. Prendergast, P. Fenner, & S. Krystal, (Eds.). *The sacred mirror: Nondual wisdom and psychotherapy* (pp. 268-289). St. Paul, Minnesota: Paragon House, p. 269.

24. Jung, C. G. (1960b). On the nature of the psyche. (R.F.C. Hull, Trans.). In H. Read, M. Fordham, & G. Adler (Eds.), *Collected works of C. G. Jung* (Vol 8, pp.159-234). New York, NY: Pantheon Books, Inc.. (Original work published in 1946).

25. Fox, M. (1999). *Sins of the spirit, blessings of the flesh*, p. 105.

26. Miller, A. (1990) *Bannished knowledge: Facing childhood injuries.* (L. Vennewitz, Trans.) New York: Doubleday, p. 109.

27. Ibid., p. 38.

28. Disque, J. G. & Bitter, J. R. (2004, Summer). Emotion, experience, and early recollections: Exploring restorative reorientation processes in Adlerian therapy. *The Journal of Individual Psychology*, 60, 115-131.

29. Miller, R. (2003). Welcoming all that is: Nonduality, Yoga Nidra, and the play of opposites in psychotherapy. In J. Prendergast, P. Fenner, & S. Krystal, (Eds.). *The sacred mirror: Nondual wisdom and psychotherapy* (pp. 209-228), p. 224.

30. Ibid.

31. Ibid.

32. Ibid.

Chapter 6

1. Rogers, C.A. (1980). *A way of being.* New York: Houghton Mifflin Company, P. 210.

2. Gendlin, E. T. (1981). *Focusing*, p. 35.

3. Hannah, B. (1981). *Encounters with the soul: Active imagination as developed by C.G. Jung.* Boston, MA: Sigo Press.

4. Bodian, S. (2002). Deconstructing the Self: The uses of inquiry in psychotherapy and spiritual practice. In J. Prendergast, P. Fenner, & S. Krystal, (Eds.). *The sacred mirror: Nondual wisdom and psychotherapy* (pp. 229-248), p. 241.

5. Ibid.

6. Jung, C. G. (1961). *Memories, dreams, reflections.* (Winston, C. and Winston, R., Trans.). NY: Vintage Books, p. 179.

7. Perls, F. (1969). *Gestalt therapy verbatim.* Lafayette, California: The Real People Press, p. 23.

8. Prendergast, J. (2003a). Introduction. In J. Prendergast, P. Fenner, & S. Krystal, (Eds.). *The sacred mirror: Nondual wisdom and psychotherapy* (pp. 1-22), p. 16.

9. Krystal, S. (2003). A nondual approach to EMDR: Psychotherapy as satsang. In J. Prendergast, P. Fenner, & S. Krystal, (Eds.). *The sacred mirror: Nondual wisdom and psychotherapy* (pp. 116-137), p. 126.

10. Ibid.

11. Hunt, D. (2003). Being intimate with what is: Healing the pain of separation. In J. Prendergast, P. Fenner, & S. Krystal, (Eds.). *The sacred mirror: Nondual wisdom and psychotherapy* (pp. 164-184*).*

12. Krystal, S. (2003). A nondual approach to EMDR: Psychotherapy as satsang. In J. Prendergast, P. Fenner, & S. Krystal, (Eds.*). The sacred mirror: Nondual wisdom and psychotherapy* (pp. 116-137), p.126.

13. Ibid., 118.

14. Ibid.

15. Prendergast, J. (2003b). The sacred mirror: Being together. In J. Prendergast, P. Fenner, & S. Krystal, (Eds.). *The sacred mirror: Nondual wisdom and psychotherapy* (pp. 89-115), p.89.

16. Prendergast, J. (2003a). Introduction. In J. Prendergast, P. Fenner, & S. Krystal, (Eds.). *The sacred mirror: Nondual wisdom and psychotherapy* (pp. 1-22), p. 13.

17. Otto, R. (1923, first published in 1917 as *Das Heilige*). *The idea of the holy*. Oxford University Press. Jung later used the word numinous.

Chapter 8

1. Gershon, Michael D., M. D., (1998). *The second brain: Your gut has a mind of its own*, pp. xiv-xv.

2. Ibid, p. 236.

3. Eliot, Lise, (1999). *What's going on in there? How the Brain and mind develop in the first five years of life*. New York: Bantam Books, p. 23.

4. Latourette, K. S. (1953). *A history of Christianity*. Harper & Brothers, New York, N.Y.

Chapter 10

1. Eliot, Lise, (1999). *What's going on in there? How the Brain and mind develop in the first five years of life*. p. 23.

2. Hillman, J. (1996). *The soul's code: In search of character and calling*. New York: Warner Books.

3. Smith, M. C & Sterling, R. W. (1976), *Borne of the human family*, printed as a text for authors' Behavioral-Science Classes by Santa Fe Community College, Gainesville, FL, pp. 46-50. Smith is previous married name of author Love, M.C.

4. Ibid., pp. 167-169.

5. Ibid.

6. Rogers, C. (1961). *On becoming a person: A therapist's view of psychotherapy*, pp. 192-193.

Chapter 11

1. Grabmeier, J. (1995). *Study finds link between stress, immune system, immune system in cancer.* The Ohio State University Research News, written February 10, 1995. May be accessed in full from: http://researchnews.osu.edu/archive/apastre1.htm .

2. *Berg, J.M., Tymoczko, J.L., and Stryer, L. (2002)* Major-histocompatibility-complex proteins present peptide antigens on cell surfaces for recognition by T-cell receptors in *Biochemistry*. Section 33.5, 5th edition. New York: W H Freeman.

3. Jung, C. G. (1959). Psychological types. In V. Laszlo (Ed.), *The basic writings of C. G. Jung.* (R. F. Hull, Trans.). New York: Random House. (Original work published 1938*).*

4. Jones, D.S., Hofmann, L. and Quinn, S. (2009). *21st Century medicine: A new model for medical education and practice.* Gig Harbor, WA.

5. Ibid.

6. *Berg, J.M., Tymoczko, J.L., and Stryer, L. (2002).)* Major-histocompatibility-complex proteins present peptide antigens on cell surfaces for recognition by T-cell receptors in *Biochemistry*. Section 33.5, 5th edition. New York: W H Freeman.

7. Olson, G. (1998). Dolls, protection, healing, power, and pla*y. Somatics Magazine-Journal of The Mind/Body Arts and Sciences*, Volume XI Number 4. Dr. Geri Olson, second term chair of the Sonoma State University Psychology Department, has facilitated the Doll Project with both adults and children in making over 2000 dolls as a depth process to gain self-awareness, a positive self-image, and an in-depth understanding of the human figure. Since making art is a somatic process (felt in the body), the making of the doll brings deep somatic awareness of what it means to be human and allows the unconscious to speak through the making of

the doll to bring self-awareness to the individual. Dr. Olson is still engaged in her Doll Project to this date.

DEFINITIONS OF SOME TERMS USED

We find it important for us to define terms, as we have been using them, in our presentation of the functional use of the enteric nervous system. While the meanings of the words are quite clearly applicable in external environments, in situations in systems we constantly encounter in the outside world, we are not accustomed to relating and applying them to our internal life systems. We think some work on these terms will help us all to understand the new image of humanity we are presenting.

The first term that may be mystifying is the word *feedback*. Feedback, as used in our work, is the part of essential intelligence relevant to a system's efficient operation, which is captured over time and returned to the system during its operation to make it more reliable—to stabilize it and make a system function according to its design.

A valuable, well-known example is the system of the automobile. It is structured as an intelligent design for a purpose but it is of no use without some present and past intelligence to make it function as designed—the intelligent feedback of a driver. There seems to be very few if any systems, designed by humans, which have not, perhaps subconsciously, been copies of nature's concept of feedback. The computer would be our second choice.

It must have taken nature multi-millions of experimental failures to arrive at the idea of feedback design, and all we have to do to discover the idea of feedback is, pay attention to our bodies and copy it.

For a second set of easy to confuse terms we use, which may need clarification, are our use of the terms, *Control and Acceptance*. The image evoked by the word Control has the ancient necessity of the protection for the animal, its survival seems to have required decision-making intelligence when faced by danger as whether to flee or fight. Over time, danger has changed to a more complex form and in such a manner in more social encounters to be hardly recognizable. It now seems necessary for the human animal to retain the original previous functional purpose, but also, to be able to utilize highly developed intuitive skills to save its life or even get what it needs or wants.

This leads to a second use we have for the meaning of Control; the conscious, learned skill of control (Self-Control). It is in arena of social intercourse that the skill of self-control is developed and balanced with the success of getting the wants and necessities of life without being 'rejected'. We can test the exercise of taking too much control at the risk being rejected by another. Or, we can learn the consequence of over-control of a situation and be rejected, then modify our behavior toward more acceptability. We suggest that a child who is given freedom to experience this—trial and results—process in a non-judgmental environment from birth to middle school, will have learned to modify his interpersonal behavior and have a more successful social life with a more positive image of himself.

The other end of this teeter-totter is of course Acceptance (Self-Acceptance). This can be interpreted as Self-Concept or Self-Image. In order to achieve a positive self-image (feeling good about myself), it seems necessary that we receive acceptance from as many external sources as possible. For acceptance to be experienced, it is necessary for us to regulate self-control to receive acceptance. It seems that this process leads us to the best of friends. Once that depth of friendship is experienced, feedback of our behavior is regulated in advance, to preserve the friendship. It is then unthinkable to do anything to destroy that friendship. It seems that this is the direct path to and involves the consideration of human sexuality. However, the subject of sexuality deserves a separate discussion relative to an otherwise empty or full life. In our early work with students in the 1970s, we originally viewed the issue of over-emphasis related to sex as the *red flag of emptiness*.

Similar *red flags of emptiness*, are the human situations of pervasive distortions, used to seek and maintain control over others, for profit, power, for personal gain, or a practice of arbitrary and exclusive standards of acceptance. Such distortions seem to be used as substitutes for meaning in those humans whose lives are empty, and live in fear of meaningful human relationships. Thus these are signs of the empty/full feeling equation usually relating to early destructive, judgmental, childhood environments that could not furnish the instinctive needs of freedom to learn social strengths and experience acceptance while the child was engaged in the tangential struggle of the learning process.

The use of the *Empty/Full* feeling terms defines for us the *voice* of the inner feeling intelligence—the enteric nervous system. The 'loudest sounds the gut speaks' are familiar to everyone who has eaten a satisfying meal that suggests the upper brain goes to sleep, or has been so hungry that the upper brain was unable to think about anything else but food. There are 'softer sounds', which we tend to ignore simply because the present image of ourselves does not include the gut as a source of intelligence—and we might erroneously think, "The gut doesn't have anything to say."

We likened the empty/full concept to the automobile fuel gage. The image of the gas tank gage suggests less intense moments than actually empty or actually full. The gut voice gets louder as the gas gage approaches the empty end and thus we pay more attention to it; and we feel more comfortable if we add even a small amount of gas to the tank. If we fill the tank then we can forget it for the now—a full feeling from the gut. The gut gauge responds as does the tank gauge, to incremental changes from the empty or the full end, to warn the consciousness of the prospects in the now and on into the future, which is a subtle example of feedback.

We do not need to define the term sexuality, for sexual stimulation seems to have the comparative voice of an elephant or that of a jackass. The electrochemistry is available and the voice gets ever louder if there is nothing else important to occupy the mind. Most of us have experienced having a commitment to a stimulating interest, an occupation or disturbance of the upper brain that, at least temporarily empties the brain of sexual interest. Sexual acceptance seems to be the ultimate experience in acceptance in order to assure the future of the animal species. This assurance seems to be a factor in all life's systems, perhaps to maintain the a balance of all forms of life, to keep all the successful current experiments alive, furnished with their needs—food, air, water minerals, etc… Who knows what?

While experience with control, incrementally leads to Self-Control, experience with attention incrementally leads to total acceptance and Self-Esteem and ultimately, a new member of the species. Variations of this pattern seem to be a universal quality of all life-animal, vegetable, and mineral. If not a new member of the species, or a needed growth experience, the reward is an intimate friend with whom to improve your life, which is another example of external feedback. The System works! If Life's System did not work, the System of the Universe would not be working either, for we are an integral part of that system.

REFERENCES

Abo, T. and Hillyer, K. T. (2007). *Your immune revolution.* Kokoro Publishing.

Beck, M. (2011). Our Buddies, Our selves. *The Oprah Magazine.* Volume 12, Number 81, pp 114-119.

Berg, J.M., Tymoczko, J.L., and Stryer, L. (2002). Major-histocompatibility-complex proteins present peptide antigens on cell surfaces for recognition by T-cell receptors in *Biochemistry.* Section 33.5, 5th edition. New York: W H Freeman.

Bodian, S. (2002). Deconstructing the Self: The uses of inquiry in psychotherapy and spiritual practice. In J. Prendergast, P. Fenner, & S. Krystal, (Eds.). *The sacred mirror: Nondual wisdom and psychotherapy* (pp. 229-248). St. Paul, Minnesota: Paragon House.

Bowlby, J. (1988). *A secure base: Clinical applications of attachment theory.* London: Routledge.

Bowlby, J. (1999, first published in 1969). *Attachment,* 2nd edition, Attachment and Loss Vol. 1, New York: Basic Books.

Campbell, J. (1976, first published 1959). *The Masks of God: Primitive mythology.* New York: Penguin.

Conger, J. P. (1988). *Jung and Reich: The body as shadow.* Berkeley, CA: North Atlantic Books.

Disque, J. G. & Bitter, J. R. (2004, Summer). Emotion, experience, and early recollections: Exploring restorative reorientation processes in Adlerian therapy. *The Journal of Individual Psychology*, 60, 115-131.

Eckberg, M. (2000). *Victims of cruelty: Somatic psychology in the treatment of posttraumatic stress disorder.* Berkeley, CA: North Atlantic Books.

Encyclopedia Britannica (1958 edition), *Renaissance*, Vol. 19, pp 222-223.

Eliot, Lise, (1999). *What's going on in there? How the brain and mind develop in the first five years of life.* New York, NY: Bantam Books.

Farber, B., Brink, D., & Raskin, P. (1996). *The psychotherapy of Carl Rogers: Cases and commentary.* New York: Guilford Press.

Feldenkrais, M. (1972). *Awareness through movement: Health exercises for personal growth.* New York: Harper and Row.

Fox, M. (1999). *Sins of the spirit, blessings of the flesh.* New York, New York: Harmony Books.

Gendlin, E. T. (1981). *Focusing* (2nd ed.). New York: Bantam Books.

Gershon, M. D. (1998). *The second brain: Your gut has a mind of its own.* New York, NY: Harper Collins.

Goleman, D. (1995*). Emotional intelligence.* New York, NY: Bantam Books.

Grabmeier, J. (1995). *Study finds link between stress, immune system, immune system in cancer.* The Ohio State University Research News, written February 10, 1995. May be accessed in full from: http://researchnews.osu.edu/archive/apastre1.htm .

Hannah, B. (1981). *Encounters with the soul: Active imagination as developed by C.G. Jung.* Boston, MA: Sigo Press.

Henderson, J. L. (1967). *Thresholds of initiation.* Middletown, Connecticut: Wesleyan University Press.

Hillman, J. (1996). *The soul's code: In search of character and calling.* New York: Warner Books.

Holt, J. (1967). *How children learn.* New York: Pitman Publishing Corporation.

Hunt, D. (2003). Being intimate with what is: Healing the pain of separation. In J. Prendergast, P. Fenner, & S. Krystal, (Eds.). *The sacred mirror: Nondual wisdom and psychotherapy* (pp. 164-184*)*.

Janoe, E. & Janoe, B. (1979). Dealing with feelings via real recollections. In H. A. Olson (Ed.), *Early recollections: Their use in diagnosis and psychotherapy*. Springfield, IL: Charles C. Thomas Publisher.

Johnson, R. A. (1986). *Inner work: Using dreams and active imagination for personal growth*. San Francisco, CA: Harper.

Jones, D.S., Hofmann, L. and Quinn, S. (2009). *21st Century Medicine: A new model for medical education and practice.* Gig Harbor, WA. Downloadable from: http://www.functionalmedicine.org/ifm_ecommerce/Pro ductDetails.aspx?ProductID=174.

Jung, C. G. (1959). Psychological types. In V. Laszlo (Ed.), *The basic writings of C. G. Jung.* (R. F. Hull, Trans.). New York: Random House. (Original work published 1938).

Jung, C. G. (1960a). Instinct and the unconscious. (R.F.C. Hull, Trans.). In H. Read, M. Fordham, & G. Adler (Eds.), *Collected works of C. G. Jung* (Vol 8, pp.129-138). New York, NY: Pantheon Books, Inc.. (Original work published in 1919).

Jung, C. G. (1960b). A review of the complex theory. (R.F.C. Hull, Trans.). In H. Read, M. Fordham, & G. Adler (Eds.), *Collected works of C. G. Jung* (Vol 8, pp. 92-104). New York, NY: Pantheon Books, Inc.. (Original work published in 1946).

Jung, C. G. (1969). Conscious, unconscious, and individuation. (R.F.C. Hull, Trans.). In H. Read, M. Fordham, & G. Adler (Eds.), *Collected works of C. G. Jung* (Vol 9, pp. 275-289). New York, NY: Pantheon Books, Inc., (Original work published in 1939).

Jung, C. G. (1992). Abstracts of the Collected Works of C. G. Jung. In C. L. Rothgeb and S. M. Clemens (Eds.), *Collected Works of C. G. Jung* (Vol. 9, part 1). Karnac Books: London, UK, (Originally published in 1968).

Kohut, H. (1977). *The restoration of the self.* New York, NY: International Universities Press.

Krystal, S. (2003). A nondual approach to EMDR: Psychotherapy as satsang. In J. Prendergast, P. Fenner, & S. Krystal, (Eds.). *The sacred mirror: Non-dual wisdom and psychotherapy* (pp. 116-137). St. Paul, Minnesota: Paragon House.

Laird, J. & Bresler, C. (1990). William James and the mechanisms of emotional experience. *Personality and Social Psychology Bulletin*, 16(4), pp. 636-651.

Lao Tsu, (1972). *Tao Te Ching.* (G. Feng & J. English, Trans.) New York, NY: Vintage Books. (Original work published in 6th century B. C.)

Latourette, K. S. (1953). *A history of Christianity.* New York, NY: Harper and Brothers.

Levine, P. A. (1997). *Waking the tiger: Healing trauma.* Berkeley, CA: North Atlantic Books.

Love, S. (2007). Using somatic awareness as a guide for making healthy life choices. *Somatics Magazine-Journal Of The Mind/Body Arts and Sciences,* Volume XV, Number 2. (Silver Love is same person as author Martha C. Love)

Love, S. (2008). Healing the trauma of the body/mind split through accessing instinctual gut feelings: A protocol for facilitating the somatic reflection process (SRP). *Somatics Magazine-Journal of The Mind/Body Arts and Sciences,* Volume XV, Number 4. (Silver Love is same person as author Martha C. Love)

Maslow, A. H. (1968). *Toward a psychology of being.* New York, NY: D. Van Nostrand Company.

McCabe, L. (2004). *Depth inquiry: Qualitative investigation of self-experience.* Unpublished manuscript.

Miller, A. (1990*) Bannished knowledge: Facing childhood injuries.* (L. Vennewitz, Trans.) New York, NY: Doubleday.

Miller, R. (2003). Welcoming all that is: Nonduality, Yoga Nidra, and the play of opposites in psychotherapy. In J. Prendergast, P. Fenner, & S. Krystal, (Eds.). *The sacred mirror: Nondual wisdom and psychotherapy* (pp. 209-228). St. Paul, Minnesota: Paragon House.

Myers, I. B. (1962). *The Myers-Briggs Type Indicator*: *Manual* 1962. Princeton, NJ: Educational Testing Services.

Myers, I. B. (1980). Gifts differing. Palo Alto, CA: Consulting Psychologist Press.

Nietzsche, F. (1999, originally published in 1911). *Thus spake Zarathustra.* (T. Common, Trans.). Mineola, NY: Dover Publications, Inc.

Olson, G. (1998). Dolls, protection, healing, power, and play. *Somatics Magazine-Journal of The Mind/Body Arts and Sciences*, Volume XI, Number 4.

Otto, R. (1923, first published in 1917 as *Das Heilige*). *The idea of the holy.* Oxford University Press.

Prendergast, J. (2003a). Introduction. In J. Prendergast, P. Fenner, & S. Krystal, (Eds.). *The sacred mirror: Nondual wisdom and psychotherapy* (pp. 1-22). St. Paul, Minnesota: Paragon House.

Prendergast, J. (2003b). The sacred mirror: Being together. In J. Prendergast, P. Fenner, & S. Krystal, (Eds.). *The sacred mirror: Nondual wisdom and psychotherapy* (pp. 89-115). St. Paul, Minnesota: Paragon House.

Perera, S. (1981). *Descent to the goddess*. Toronto: Inner City Press.

Perls, F. (1969). *Gestalt therapy verbatim*. Lafayette, California,: The Real People Press.

Reiche, E.M.V., S. O. V. Numes, and H.K. Morimoto (2004). Stress, depression, the immune system, and cancer. *Lancet Oncology* 5, Number 10, pp 617-25.

Rogers, Carl R. (1961). *On becoming a person*. Massachusetts: Riverdale Press.

Rogers, C.A. (1980). *A way of being*. New York: Houghton Mifflin Company.

Servan-Schreiber, D., (2004). *The instinct to heal: Curing stress, anxiety, and depression without drugs and without talk therapy*. Emmaus, PA: Rodale, Inc.

Servan-Schreiber, D., (2008). *Anticancer: A new way of life.* New York: Viking Penguin.

Smith, M. C & Sterling, R.W. (1975), *Impact of experience*: *Access to self-awareness and organismic purpose.* Unpublished manuscript. Smith is previous married name of author Martha C. Love

Smith, M. C & Sterling, R. W. (1976), *Borne of the human family*, printed as a text for Behavioral-Science Classes by Santa Fe Community College, Gainesville, FL. Smith is previous married name of author Martha C. Love.

Stein, M. (1998). *Jung's map of the soul.* Chicago: Open Court.

Storr, A. (Ed.). (1983). *The essential Jung.* New York: MJF Books.

Taylor, J. (1983). Dream work: Techniques for discovering the creative power in dreams. NJ: Paulist Press.

Van der Kolk, B. A. , Mcfarlane, A. C., & L. (Eds.) (1996). *Traumatic stress: The effects of overwhelming experience on the mind, body, and society.* New York: Guilford Press.

Viscottt, D. (1990). *The language of feeling.* New York: Pocket Books.

Viscott, D. (1992). *Emotionally Free: Letting go of the past to live in the moment.* Chicago, IL: Contemporary Books.

Weis, R. (1973) *Loneliness: The experience of emotional and social isolation.* Cambridge, MA: The Massachusetts Institute of Technology.

Winnicott, D. W. (1965). From dependence to independence in the development of the individual. In *The maturational process and the facilitating environment* (pp. 83-99). New York: International Universities Press (Original work published 1963).

Winnicott, D. W. (1971). *Playing and reality.* New York: Penguin Books.

Winton, W. (1990). Jameian aspects of misattribution research. *Personality and Social Psychology Bulletin,* 16(4), pp. 652-664.

Wittine, B. (2003). Jungian analysis and nondual wisdom. In J. Prendergast, P. Fenner, & S. Krystal, (Eds.). *The sacred mirror: Nondual wisdom and psychotherapy* (pp. 268-289). St. Paul, Minnesota: Paragon House.

Woodman, M. (1982). *Addiction to perfection.* Toronto, Canada: Inner City Books.

Woodman, M. & Mellick, J. (2000). *Coming home to myself: Reflections for nurturing a woman's body and soul.* Boston, MA: Conai Press.

Yogananda, P. (1983). *Songs of the soul.* L.A., CA: International Publications Council of Self-Realization.

ABOUT THE AUTHORS

Martha Char (Silver) Love, MA in Educational Psychology, MA in Depth (Analytical) Psychology, PMA in Art Therapy
email: silver_love_@hotmail.com

Robert W. (Bob) Sterling, BSEE in Electrical Engineering, MRE in Religious Education
email: sterlingrwalter@gmail.com

While working as colleagues together at Santa Fe Community College, Gainesville, Florida, in the 1970s, we accepted the tasks of teaching and operating a Career Guidance and Assessment Program (Career GAP) that served both the community college students and as a storefront for the general population. Silver had experienced the impact of growing up in the South in the '50s and early '60s, and came equipped with a degree in Elementary Education and a Master's degree in Educational Psychology with a license in School Psychology. Bob was raised in Northern Ohio, carrying the direct impact of WWII in Europe, with an Electrical Engineering degree, a Masters in Religious Education, and Industrial experience in Electronics. The convergence of our two personalities and experiences of our own personal traumas enabled us to critically look at and question what was happening in counseling methodology, particularly when dealing with a wide variety of social problems. It is from this initial work that this book is based.

Since that time and for the past 35 years, both of us have continued to work and study independently in the field of education and psychology, always exploring the awareness of the instinctual gut response and how this awareness might paint a new image of human nature. In 2005, we began sharing our independent studies and new clinical research work together once again (thanks to the internet and email). With Dr. Michael Gershon's recent neurological breakthrough identifying the gut brain, we were inspired to write this book as an account of our life's work exploring the psychology of gut intelligence, and what that means about human nature and the future of our species.

CPSIA information can be obtained at www.ICGtesting.com
Printed in the USA
LVOW05s1950121114

413338LV00034B/2203/P